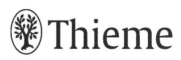

Oral Cancer Surgery: A Visual Guide

Marco Kesting, MD, DMD, FEBOMFS, Priv.-Doz.
Department of Oral and Maxillofacial Surgery
Klinikum Rechts der Isar, University of Technology
Munich, Germany

208 illustrations

Thieme
Stuttgart • New York • Delhi • Rio

Library of Congress Cataloging-in-Publication Data

Kesting, Marco, author.
  Oral cancer surgery : a visual guide / Marco Kesting.
     p. ; cm.
  Includes bibliographical references.
    ISBN 978-3-13-199401-1 (hardback : alk. paper) – ISBN 978-3-13-199411-0 (e-book)
  I. Title.
  [DNLM: 1. Oral Surgical Procedures–methods–Atlases. 2. Mouth Neoplasms–surgery–Atlases. WU 600.7]
  RD662
  616.99'431059–dc23
                                                    2014023170

© 2015 Georg Thieme Verlag KG

Thieme Publishers Stuttgart
Rüdigerstrasse 14, 70469 Stuttgart, Germany
+49 [0]711 8931 421, customerservice@thieme.de

Thieme Publishers New York
333 Seventh Avenue, New York, NY 10001 USA
+1 800 782 3488, customerservice@thieme.com

Thieme Publishers Delhi
A-12, Second Floor, Sector-2, Noida-201301
Uttar Pradesh, India
+91 120 45 566 00, customerservice@thieme.in

Thieme Publishers Rio, Thieme Publicações Ltda.
Argentina Building 16th floor, Ala A, 228 Praia do Botafogo
Rio de Janeiro 22250-040 Brazil
+55 21 3736-3631

Cover design: Thieme Publishing Group
Typesetting by DiTech Process Solutions, India

Printed in China by Everbest Printing Ltd   5 4 3 2 1

ISBN 978-3-13-199401-1

Also available as an e-book:
eISBN 978-3-13-199411-0

Important note: Medicine is an ever-changing science undergoing continual development. Research and clinical experience are continually expanding our knowledge, in particular our knowledge of proper treatment and drug therapy. Insofar as this book mentions any dosage or application, readers may rest assured that the authors, editors, and publishers have made every effort to ensure that such references are in accordance with **the state of knowledge at the time of production of the book.**

Nevertheless, this does not involve, imply, or express any guarantee or responsibility on the part of the publishers in respect to any dosage instructions and forms of applications stated in the book. **Every user is requested to examine carefully** the manufacturers' leaflets accompanying each drug and to check, if necessary in consultation with a physician or specialist, whether the dosage schedules mentioned therein or the contraindications stated by the manufacturers differ from the statements made in the present book. Such examination is particularly important with drugs that are either rarely used or have been newly released on the market. Every dosage schedule or every form of application used is entirely at the user's own risk and responsibility. The authors and publishers request every user to report to the publishers any discrepancies or inaccuracies noticed. If errors in this work are found after publication, errata will be posted at www.thieme.com on the product description page.

Some of the product names, patents, and registered designs referred to in this book are in fact registered trademarks or proprietary names even though specific reference to this fact is not always made in the text. Therefore, the appearance of a name without designation as proprietary is not to be construed as a representation by the publisher that it is in the public domain.

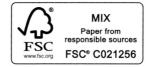

Inter omnes partes medicinae chirurgiae effectus evidentissimus

–Aulus Cornelius Celsus (Roman encyclopaedist)

Contents

Preface ix

Acknowledgments x

1   Airway Management 1

1.1	**Tracheotomy** 2	1.2	**Technique of Tracheotomy** 4
1.1.1	History 2		
1.1.2	Relevant Anatomy for Tracheotomy 3		

2   Lymph Node Management 9

2.1   **General Overview of Neck Dissection** 10
2.1.1   History 10
2.1.2   Classification and Clinical Management 10
2.1.3   Relevant Anatomy of the Neck 11
2.1.4   Definition and Description of the Cervical Lymph Node Groups: Levels and Sublevels of the Neck. 12

2.2   **Neck Dissection Levels I to III (Supraomohyoid Dissection)** 15
2.2.1   Preliminary Considerations and Recommended Procedure 15

2.2.2   Technique of Neck Dissection Levels I to III .. 16

2.3   **Neck Dissection Levels IV and V** 25
2.3.1   Preliminary Considerations and Recommended Approaches 25
2.3.2   Relevant Anatomy for Level V Dissection 26
2.3.3   Technique of Posterior Neck Dissection (MacFee Approach). 27
2.3.4   Alternative Approaches for Levels I to V 26

3   Ablative Tumor Surgery 33

3.1   **Access to the Tumor and Tumor Resection** 34
3.1.1   Overview and Accessibility 34
3.1.2   Alternative Approaches and Indications 34

3.2   **Lip-split Mandibulotomy Access** 34
3.2.1   History 34
3.2.2   Modifications 35
3.2.3   Technique 36

3.3   **Weber-Fergusson-Dieffenbach Approach** 41
3.3.1   History 41
3.3.2   Technique 41

3.4   **Midfacial Degloving** 43

3.4.1   History 43
3.4.2   Technique 43

3.5   **Le-Fort-I Osteotomy Approach** 46
3.5.1   History 46
3.5.2   Technique 46

3.6   **Tumor Access: Further Approaches** 47
3.6.1   To the Upper Part of the Oral Cavity and the Midface 47
3.6.2   To the Lower Part of the Oral Cavity 47

3.7   **Tumor Resection** 48
3.7.1   Technique 48

4   Reconstructive Surgery 51

4.1   **Considerations on Reconstructive Procedures** 52

4.2   **Suggestions for Reconstructive Algorithms** 52

4.3 Nasolabial Flap 54
4.3.1 History 54
4.3.2 Flap Anatomy 54
4.3.3 Indications 55
4.3.4 Variations 55
4.3.5 Technique 55

4.4 Deltopectoral Flap 60
4.4.1 History 60
4.4.2 Flap Design and Anatomy 60
4.4.3 Indication 61
4.4.4 Technique 61

4.5 Microvascular Anastomosis 66
4.5.1 History 66
4.5.2 Technique 67

4.6 Radial Forearm Flap 70
4.6.1 History 70
4.6.2 Indication 70
4.6.3 Preliminary Examinations and Considerations 70
4.6.4 Technique 71

4.7 Anterolateral Thigh Flap/ Myocutaneous Vastus Lateralis Flap 75
4.7.1 History 75

4.7.2 Indication 75
4.7.3 Preoperative Procedures 75
4.7.4 Technique 75
4.7.5 Modification of the Procedure by Harvesting an Additional Myocutaneous Tensor Fasciae Latae Flap 83

4.8 Osseocutaneous Fibula Flap 85
4.8.1 History 85
4.8.2 Indication 85
4.8.3 Preoperative Procedures 85
4.8.4 Cross-sectional Anatomy 87
4.8.5 Technique 88

4.9 Considerable Alternatives in Reconstruction 96
4.9.1 Pedicled Flaps 96
4.9.2 Free Flaps 96

4.10 Principles of Complex Reconstruction Planning 97
4.10.1 Classification of Mandibular Defects 97
4.10.2 Mandibular Reconstruction with Osseocutaneous Fibula Flaps 98
4.10.3 Combined Mandibula and Tongue Reconstruction 115

Index 119

Preface

Operative treatment for oral cancer is one of the most challenging fields in whole surgery. The perioral region is the only area of the body containing all types of tissue: muscle, bone, cartilage, skin, and mucosa. Because of this unique anatomy, ablative tumor surgery and reconstructive surgery remain very complex. On the one hand, the surgeon has to possess elaborate skills in handling the soft tissue, dealing with microvascular techniques and managing bone treatment including osteosynthesis. On the other hand, the surgeon has to prepare defined strategies to anticipate any upcoming surgical problem. Because there is an overwhelming repertoire of ablative and reconstructive procedures, it is hard for students, residents and young surgeons to find the right way to "survive in the operative jungle."

This book concentrates on key procedures that offer young surgeons the possibility to solve almost any case of oral cancer. Basic principles are didactically edited in series of pictures and/or diagrams. Traditional approaches are combined with innovative techniques. Anatomical introductions connect previous knowledge with the surgical procedures. Additionally, historic landmarks and recommendations regarding to the techniques are given in an informational, sometimes anecdotic style. The compact and concise character of the book should enable the resident to study, prepare, and recapitulate all issues regarding oral cancer surgery in a short time.

Marco Kesting, MD, DMD, FEBOMFS, Priv.-Doz.

Acknowledgments

This book would not have been possible without the support, discussion, and advice that I received from my most highly respected and honored academic teacher, Professor Klaus-Dietrich Wolff, over all the years that we have worked together. Thanks are also due to Dr. Dr. Florian Bauer, Dr. Andreas Fichter, Dr. Aakshay Gulati, cand. med. Daniela König, Dr. Dr. Kilian Kreutzer, Ali Kurt, Priv.-Doz. Dr. Dr. Thomas Mücke, Dr. Markus Nieberler, cand. med. Christopher-Philipp Nobis, Dr. Niklas Rommel, Dr. Dr. Nils Rohleder, Priv.-Doz. Dr. Elias Scherer, and Dr. Dr. Jochen Weitz for their inspiration, contributions, and proofreading.

Chapter 1

Airway Management

1.1	Tracheotomy	2
1.2	Technique of Tracheotomy	4
	Recommended Reading	8

1

1.1 Tracheotomy

The success of oral cancer surgery depends on appropriate airway management; therefore, tracheotomy is a key procedure.

1.1.1 History

2950 to 2800 BC

The first images of a tracheotomy may date as far back as Ancient Egypt. On two stone plates dated to the first dynasty (2950–2800 BC), two people are depicted sitting or kneeling next to each other, one of them touching the upper thorax of the other with a knifelike object. Whether these images in fact depict a tracheotomy is, however, highly controversial.

128 to 60 BC

From the writings of Galen (129–199 AD), we know that Asclepiades (128–60 BC), Cicero's personal physician who practiced medicine in Rome, suggested opening the trachea as a measure of last resort to avoid asphyxiation. Via the Arab world, the knowledge of this technique was eventually brought to the Occident under the name of "subscannatio," meaning "cutting the throat."

1546

Antonio Musa Brassavola from Ferrara (1500–1555) performed and published the first documented case of a successful tracheotomy in 1546. The patient was on the verge of death from "an abscess in the windpipe."

19th Century to Today

Tracheotomy became a routine operation at the beginning of the 19th century for the treatment of diphtheria. The French physician Pierre Bretonneau (1778–1862) and his apprentice Armand Trousseau (1801–1867) established a standardized procedure, which was later adapted throughout Europe. However, this procedure was still considered controversial, as can be seen in the circumstances of George Washington's death in 1799. The first president of the United States of America presumably suffered from a severe case of laryngitis. His personal physician, who had heard of tracheotomy but had not actually performed the procedure himself, decided not to perform his first tracheotomy on a person of such high rank, instead relying on traditional techniques. George Washington died, perhaps not surprisingly, after losing about 2.5 L of blood from four bloodlettings within 12 hours. Chevalier Jackson (1865–1958), professor for laryngology at Pittsburgh University, achieved the next breakthrough in tracheotomy. He departed from the tradition of high tracheostomy, which was performed to preserve the thyroid gland and pretracheal vessels. By implementing the new technique of the "cricoid cartilage should never be cut," the problem of laryngeal stenosis was solved.

Whereas, at the beginning of the last century, tracheotomy was basically an emergency procedure used in cases of upper airway obstruction, this indication is the exception nowadays. Tracheotomy today is the most common surgical procedure performed in long-time ventilated intensive care patients.

1.1.2 Relevant Anatomy for Tracheotomy

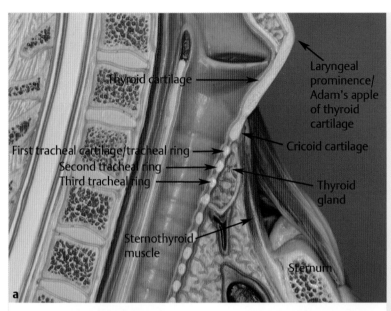

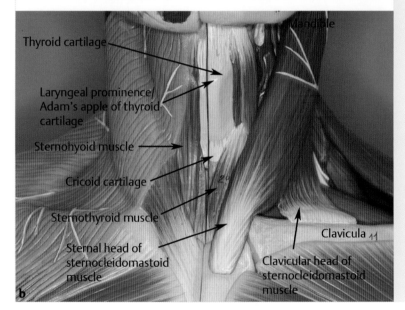

Fig. 1.1a, b Anatomy of the infrahyoid region and the jugular notch (sagittal and frontal view), shown on anatomic torso model (SOMSO, Coburg, Germany). Keep to the dogma "cricoid cartilage should never be cut" and cut between the second and the third tracheal ring.

1.2 Technique of Tracheotomy

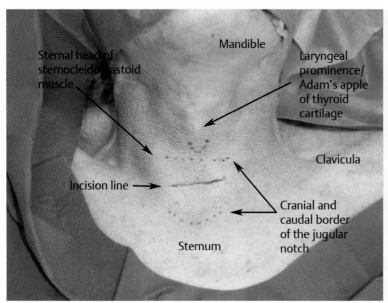

Mandible

Sternal head of sternocleidomastoid muscle

Laryngeal prominence/ Adam's apple of thyroid cartilage

Incision line

Clavicula

Cranial and caudal border of the jugular notch

Sternum

Fig. 1.2 Anatomic landmarks for skin incision. The leading landmarks are the laryngeal prominence of the thyroid cartilage and the jugular notch. The incision is made halfway between the laryngeal prominence and the caudal border of the jugular notch.

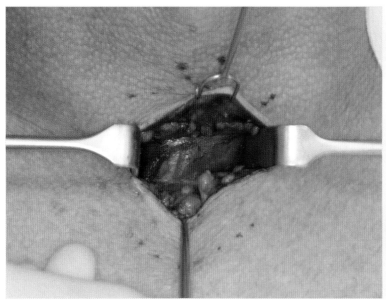

Fig. 1.3 Incision of skin, subcutaneous fatty tissue down to the sternothyroid muscle.

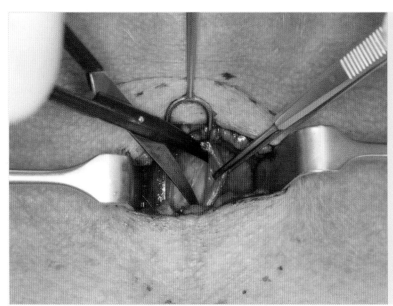

Fig. 1.4 Midline division and undermining of the sternothyroid muscle.

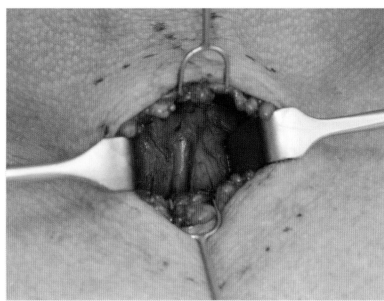

Fig. 1.5 Thyroid gland with overlying vein becomes visible.

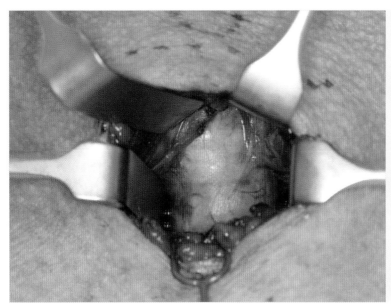

Fig. 1.6 Thyroid gland is retracted in cranial direction, trachea becomes visible.

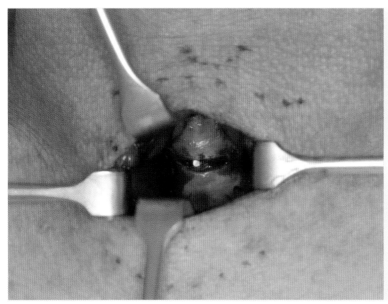

Fig. 1.7 Transverse incision of the trachea between the second and third tracheal rings.

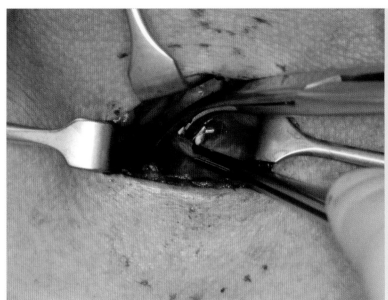

Fig. 1.8 Vertical lateral incisions of the trachea in caudal direction.

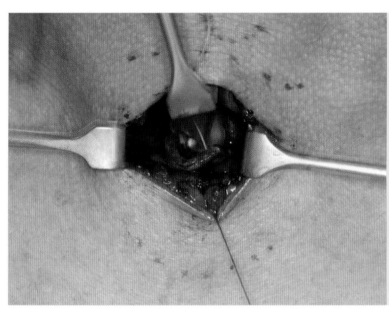

Fig. 1.9 The inversely U-shaped tracheal plate is fixed with two 2–0 Vicryl sutures (Ethicon, Somerville, NJ) to the subcutaneous tissue.

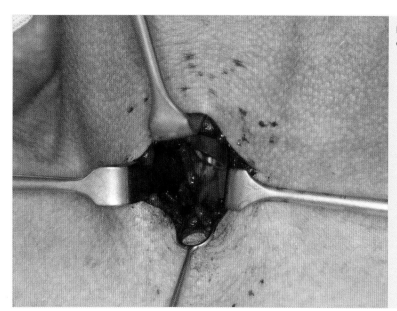

Fig. 1.10 The nasopharyngeal tube is pulled out.

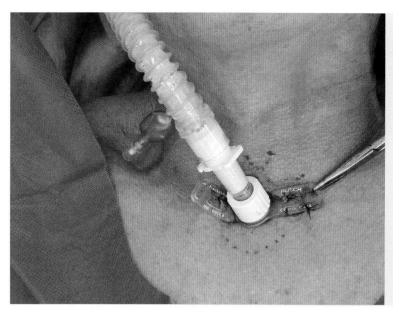

Fig. 1.11 Insertion of the tracheal tube and lateral fixation of the tracheal tube to the skin.

Recommended Reading

Alberti PW. Tracheotomy versus intubation. A 19th century controversy. Ann Otol Rhinol Laryngol 1984; 93: 333–337

Carroll CM, Pahor A. The history of tracheotomy. J Ir Coll Physicians Surg 2001; 30: 237–238

Cohen J, Stock M, Chan B et al. Microvascular reconstruction and tracheotomy are significant determinants of resource utilization in head and neck surgery. Arch Otolaryngol Head Neck Surg 2000; 126: 947–949

Frost EA. Tracing the tracheostomy. Ann Otol Rhinol Laryngol 1976; 85: 618–624

Haddad FS. Ibn Zuhr and experimental tracheostomy and tracheotomy. J Am Coll Surg 2004; 199: 665

Jackson C. Tracheotomy. Laryngoscope 1909; 19: 285–290

Jackson C. High tracheotomy and other errors: the chief causes of chronic laryngeal stenosis. Surg Gynecol Obstet 1923; 32: 392–398

Pahor AL. Ear, nose and throat in Ancient Egypt. J Laryngol Otol 1992; 106: 773–779

Pratt LW, Ferlito A, Rinaldo A. Tracheotomy: historical review. Laryngoscope 2008; 118: 1597–1606

Chapter 2

Lymph Node Management

2.1	General Overview of Neck Dissection	10
2.2	Neck Dissection Levels I to III (Supraomohyoid Dissection)	15
2.3	Neck Dissection Levels IV and V	25
	Recommended Reading	32

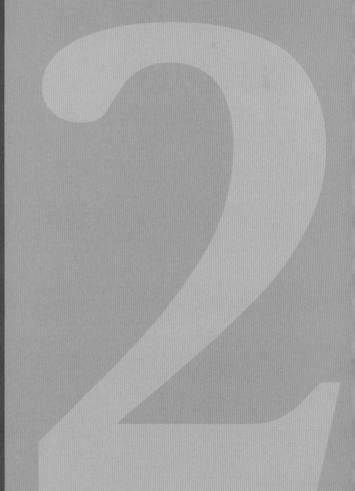

2.1 General Overview of Neck Dissection

2.1.1 History

1888

Franciszek Jawdynski (1851–1896), a surgeon from Warsaw, was the first to perform a neck dissection in metastasizing head and neck carcinomas. He described an en bloc resection of the lymph nodes together with the carotid artery, the internal jugular vein, and the sternocleidomastoid muscle; unfortunately, because his description was in Polish, it did not gain much popularity.

1906

George Washington Crile (1864–1943), from Cleveland, Ohio, described his experience with 132 cases of radical neck dissection in head and neck carcinomas.

1962

Argentinian Osvaldo Suarez (1912–1972), from Cordoba, introduced in the Spanish literature his concept of the modified neck dissection with preservation of one or more nonlymphatic structures. It was reported that he did a modified neck dissection in an astonishing 20 minutes. After some visits to Argentina, Ettore Bocca (1914–2003), from Ferrara, Italy, popularized the modified neck dissection in English language publications.

2.1.2 Classification and Clinical Management

As a basic principle, ipsilateral neck dissection of levels I to III is performed in all carcinomas of the oral cavity that have not been operated on previously. Bilateral neck dissection of levels I to III is categorically done when the intraoral malignancy extends over the midline. Neck dissection is started with dissection of the ipsilateral level II and III lymph nodes, which are immediately sent to a pathologist who performs instantaneous sections from the tissue. If lymph node metastasis is found, neck dissection is extended to levels IV and V on the ipsilateral side and levels I to III on the contralateral side.

Management of the clinical and radiological negative neck includes a functional neck dissection. Strict focus has to be paid to preserving the spinal accessory nerve (SAN), the sternocleidomastoid (SCM) muscle, and the internal jugular vein (IJV). Even in positive necks, these structures should be preserved when the lymph nodes can be dissected clearly off these structures.

Management of lymph node–positive necks with clear adherence of lymph node metastases to one of the mentioned structures includes a modified radical neck dissection. The adhered structure (SAN, SCM muscle, or IJV) has to be included in the dissection.

Management of the lymph node–positive neck with adherence of the lymph node metastasis to all three structures (SAN, SCM muscle, and IJV) includes a radical neck dissection.

There is no evidence-based clinical benefit in resecting the neck dissection specimen en bloc. Therefore, splitting the neck dissection levels in stages is preferred as shown in the following techniques of neck dissection. This approach facilitates the postoperative tumor board review discussion. The exact pinpointing of cervical metastasis for adjuvant radiotherapy is alleviated.

2.1.3 Relevant Anatomy of the Neck

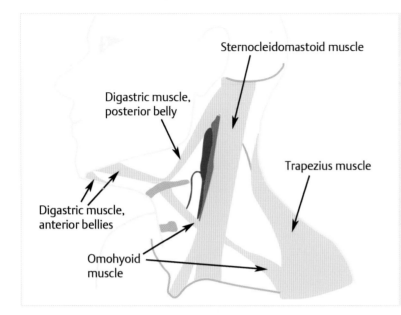

Fig. 2.1 Important muscular landmarks.

Sternocleidomastoid muscle

Digastric muscle, posterior belly

Trapezius muscle

Digastric muscle, anterior bellies

Omohyoid muscle

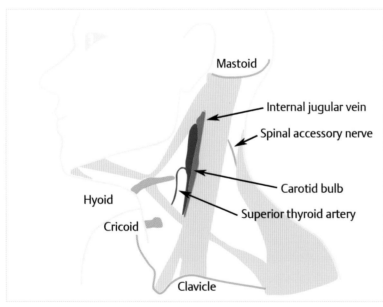

Fig. 2.2 Important vascular, nerval, and bony landmarks.

Mastoid

Internal jugular vein

Spinal accessory nerve

Carotid bulb

Superior thyroid artery

Hyoid

Cricoid

Clavicle

2.1.4 Definition and Description of the Cervical Lymph Node Groups: Levels and Sublevels of the Neck

I.   Submental and submandibular nodes
     Ia) Submental triangle
     Ib) Submandibular triangle
II. Upper jugular nodes
     IIa) Nodes located medial to the vertical plane defined by the SAN
     IIb) Nodes located lateral to the vertical plane defined by the SAN
III. Middle jugular nodes
IV. Lower jugular nodes
V.   Posterior triangle group
     Va) Nodes above the cricoid
     Vb) Nodes below the cricoid

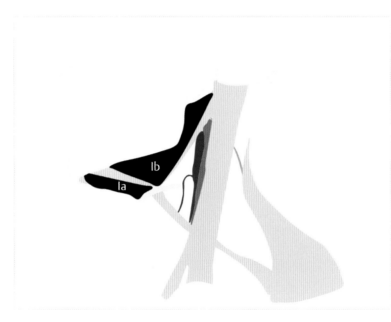

Fig. 2.3 Level I is bound by the body of the mandible superiorly, posterior belly of the digastric muscle posteriorly, and the anterior belly of the digastric muscle on the contralateral side anteriorly. Level Ia is bound by the anterior bellies of the digastric muscles laterally, by the mylohyoid at its base, and by the hyoid bone caudally. Level Ib is formed by the anterior and posterior bellies of the digastric muscle and the body of the mandible.

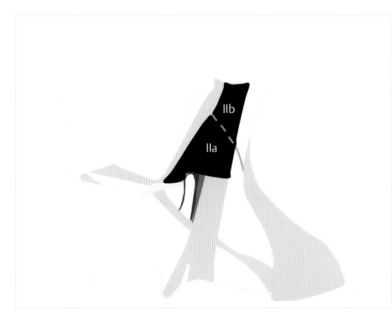

Fig. 2.4 Level II includes nodes of the upper third of the jugular vein, extending from the skull base to the inferior border of the hyoid bone. The region is defined by the digastric muscle superiorly and the hyoid bone and the carotid bifurcation inferiorly. Level II is divided into IIa and IIb by the SAN.

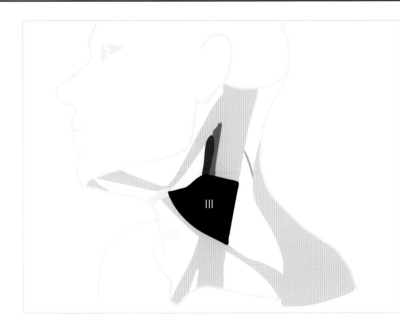

Fig. 2.5 Level III includes the middle third of the jugular nodes. The region extends from the carotid bifurcation and the hyoid bone superiorly to the omohyoid muscle inferiorly.

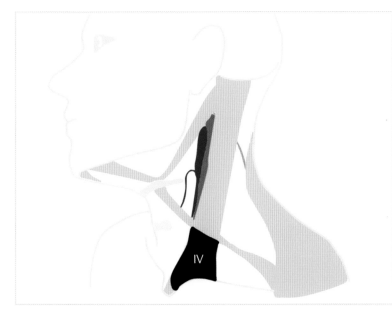

Fig. 2.6 Level IV includes lower jugular nodes extending from the omohyoid muscle superiorly to the clavicle inferiorly.

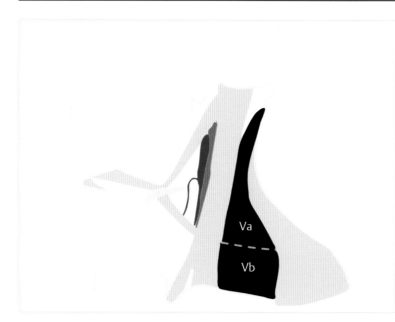

Fig. 2.7 Level V includes lymph nodes located along the lower half of the SAN and the transverse cervical artery, as well as the supraclavicular nodes. The region's posterior boundary is the anterior border of the trapezius muscle, the anterior boundary is the posterior border of the SCM muscle, and the inferior boundary is the clavicle. Level V is divided into Va and Vb by the cricoid.

2.2 Neck Dissection Levels I to III (Supraomohyoid Dissection)

2.2.1 Preliminary Considerations and Recommended Procedure

There is no evidence-based clinical benefit in resecting the neck dissection specimen en bloc. Splitting the neck dissection levels into stages A to E is therefore preferred, as illustrated in Fig. 2.8 and the following photo series "Technique of neck dissection" (Fig. 2.9 to 2.26). This approach facilitates the postoperative tumor board review discussion, especially with the pathologist. Exact pinpointing of cervical metastasis for adjuvant radiotherapy is alleviated.

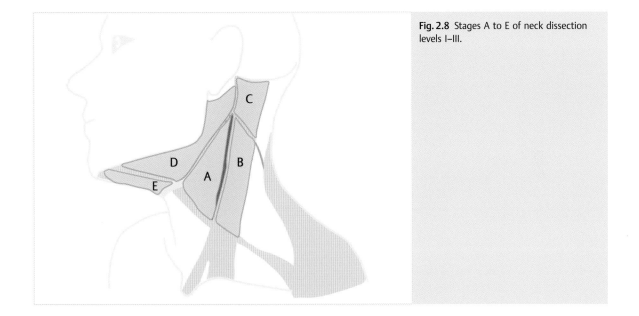

Fig. 2.8 Stages A to E of neck dissection levels I–III.

2.2.2 Technique of Neck Dissection
Levels I to III

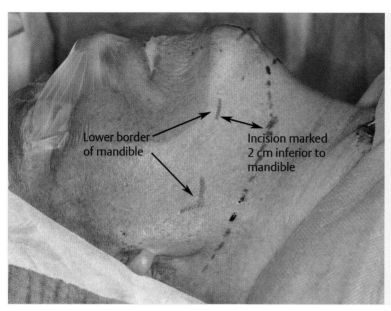

Fig. 2.9 Patient positioned with neck extended, appropriate draping, and antiseptic skin preparation. Incision line is marked 2 cm caudal to the mandibular margin.

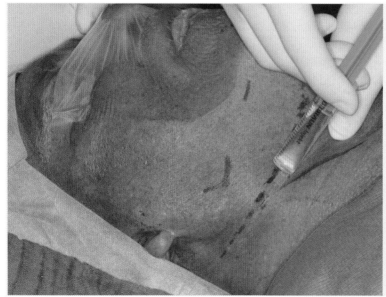

Fig. 2.10 Infiltration of 5 mL local anaesthetic with 1:200,000 adrenaline.

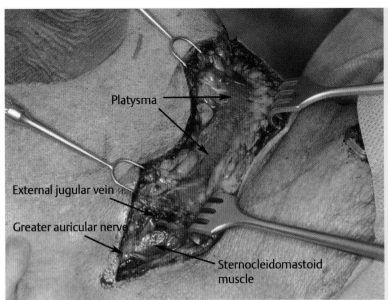

Fig. 2.11 Incision of skin and subcutaneous fatty tissue down to the platysma muscle. Posterior extent of the incision: point at which the greater auricular nerve crosses the posterior border of the SCM muscle. Anterior extent of incision: contralateral anterior belly of the digastric muscle.

Platysma

External jugular vein

Greater auricular nerve

Sternocleidomastoid muscle

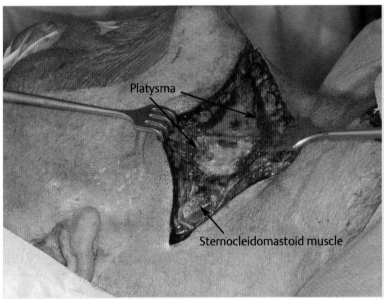

Fig. 2.12 Division of the platysma muscle and definition of the anterior margin of the SCM muscle.

Platysma

Sternocleidomastoid muscle

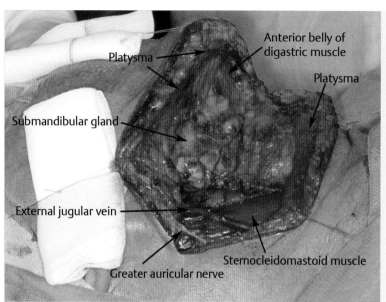

Platysma — Anterior belly of digastric muscle

Platysma

Submandibular gland

External jugular vein

Sternocleidomastoid muscle

Greater auricular nerve

Fig. 2.13 Reflection of the platysma muscle cranially and caudally. Fixation of the skin–platysma flaps with sutures superiorly and inferiorly. Exposure of the ipsilateral anterior belly of digastric muscle down to the hyoid bone.

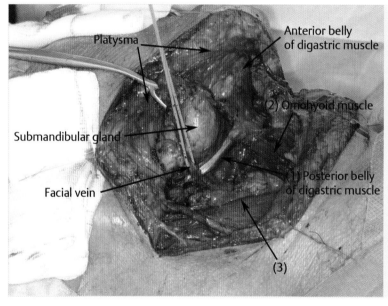

Platysma — Anterior belly of digastric muscle

(2) Omohyoid muscle

Submandibular gland

Facial vein

(1) Posterior belly of digastric muscle

(3)

Fig. 2.14 Definition of the muscle landmarks: (1) Exposure of the posterior belly of the digastric muscle in anteroposterior direction to the point at which it is crossed by the facial vein; (2) exposure of the omohyoid muscle from the hyoid bone to the point at which it reaches the SCM muscle; and (3) exposure of the anterior border of the SCM muscle from its cranial origin to the point at which it is crossed by the omohyoid muscle.

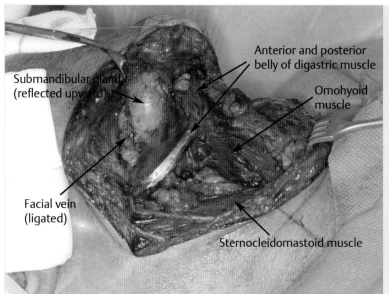

Submandibular gland
(reflected upward)

Anterior and posterior
belly of digastric muscle

Omohyoid
muscle

Facial vein
(ligated)

Sternocleidomastoid muscle

Fig. 2.15 Ligation of the facial vein and exposure of the posterior belly of the digastric muscle to the mastoid process.

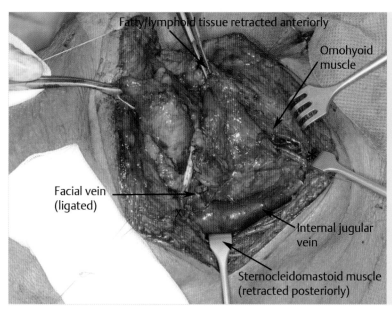

Fatty/lymphoid tissue retracted anteriorly

Omohyoid
muscle

Facial vein
(ligated)

Internal jugular
vein

Sternocleidomastoid muscle
(retracted posteriorly)

Fig. 2.16 Start removal of block A (Fig. 2.8). Facultative circumferential dissection of the IJV (lateral, anterior, and medial surfaces have to be dissected necessarily). Inferior limit of dissection of the IJV: the level of omohyoid and SCM muscle crossing (*). Superior limit of dissection of the IJV: the point at which the IJV is crossed by the posterior belly of the digastric muscle (X).

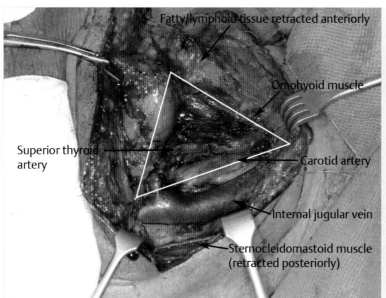

Fatty/lymphoid tissue retracted anteriorly

Omohyoid muscle

Superior thyroid artery

Carotid artery

Internal jugular vein

Sternocleidomastoid muscle (retracted posteriorly)

Fig. 2.17 Block A (Fig. 2.8)—the fatty/lymphoid tissue overlying the carotid artery and the superior thyroid artery—is removed. The tissue block is bounded by an anatomic triangle formed by the IJV, the omohyoid muscle, and the posterior belly of the digastric muscle.

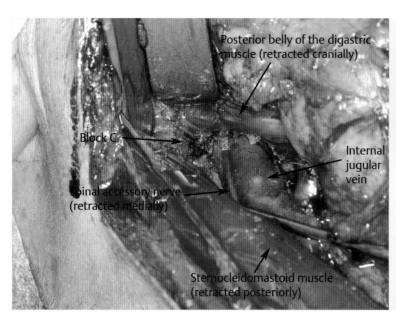

Posterior belly of the digastric muscle (retracted cranially)

Block C

Internal jugular vein

Spinal accessory nerve (retracted medially)

Sternocleidomastoid muscle (retracted posteriorly)

Fig. 2.18 Identification of the SAN, which can be found in close proximity to the meeting point of the IJV and the posterior belly of the digastric muscle. The nerve runs along the line, bisecting the right angle formed by the IJV and the posterior belly of the digastric muscle. Dissection of the SAN deep to the SCM muscle.

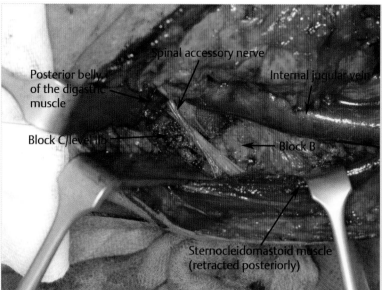

Posterior belly of the digastic muscle

Spinal accessory nerve

Internal jugular vein

Block C/level Ib

Block B

Sternocleidomastoid muscle (retracted posteriorly)

Fig. 2.19 Removal of block B (Fig. 2.8), the fatty/lymphoid tissue located caudal to the SAN, posterior of the IJV, and cranial to the crossing point of the omohyoid/SCM muscles. Removal of the fatty/lymphoid tissue located caudal to the mastoid process, cranial to the SAN, and anterior to the SCM muscle (block C, Fig. 2.8); beware of bleeding from the occipital artery.

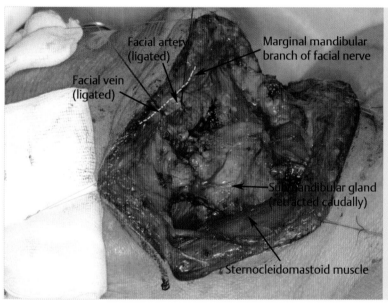

Facial artery (ligated)

Marginal mandibular branch of facial nerve

Facial vein (ligated)

Submandibular gland (retracted caudally)

Sternocleidomastoid muscle

Fig. 2.20 Ligation of the facial vein and artery (can be palpated at the mandibular margin). The mandibular marginal branch (highlighted by dotting) of the facial nerve can be protected by retracting the ligated facial vessels in a cranial direction. Dissection of the contents of the submandibular triangle (block D, Fig. 2.8) from the periosteum of the mandible.

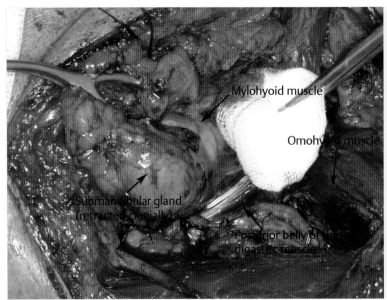

Fig. 2.21 Blunt dissection of the submandibular triangle contents from the mylohyoid muscle anteriorly and from the posterior belly of the digastric muscle caudally.

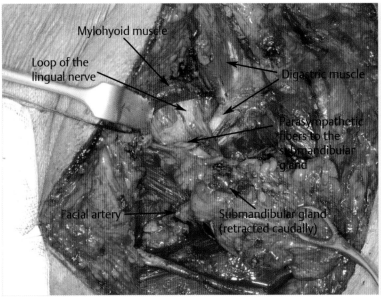

Fig. 2.22 Dissection of the loop of the lingual nerve and identification of the parasympathetic fibers to the submandibular gland.

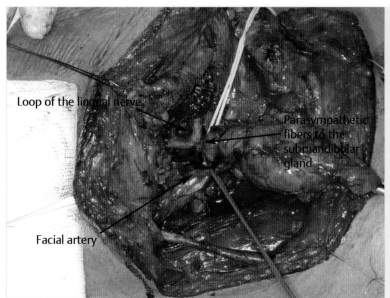

Loop of the lingual nerve

Parasympathetic fibers to the submandibular gland

Facial artery

Fig. 2.23 Parasympathetic fibers to the submandibular gland are highlighted by a yellow vessel loop. The proximally pedicled facial artery is highlighted by a red vessel loop. Ligation of both of the structures and removal of the block D (Fig. 2.8) contents.

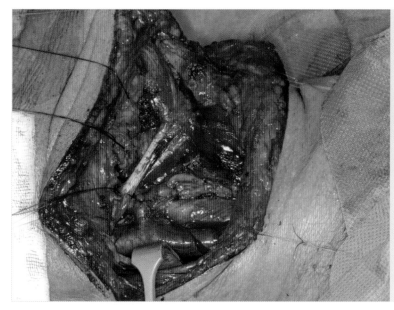

Fig. 2.24 Appearance following removal of levels Ib, II, and III (blocks A to D, Fig. 2.8) contents.

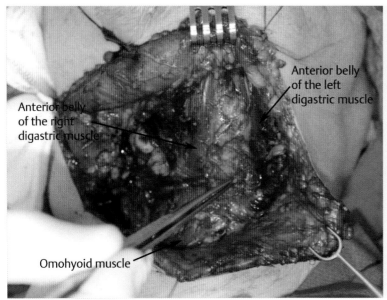

Fig. 2.25 Finally, block E (Fig. 2.8), which is located between the anterior bellies of the digastric muscles, the mylohyoid muscle, and the hyoid bone, is resected.

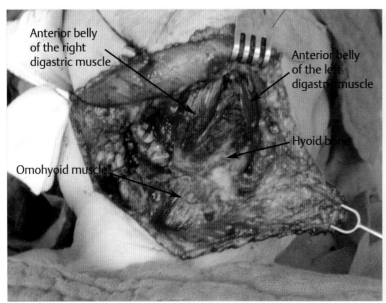

Fig. 2.26 Final appearance after resection of lymphatic and fatty tissue block E (Fig. 2.8).

2.3 Neck Dissection Levels IV and V

2.3.1 Preliminary Considerations and Recommended Approaches

- Level IV dissection is possible by gaining the same access as recommended for levels I to III; please be aware of the thoracic duct on the left side as there is limited access in the caudal region.
- The horizontal access to levels I to III generally allows two variations for extended access to level IV and V nodes: MacFee and a modified Schobinger approach (Fig. 2.27).

- Irradiated neck: the MacFee approach leads to less wound healing disturbances.
- Modified Schobinger incision: better access to the posterior triangle and the complete course of the accessory nerve.
- Modified Schobinger incision: angle of the cranioposterior tip has to be at least 90°; therefore, take care that the posterior incision for the level I to III dissection is not extended cranially to the mastoid/ear lobe region—otherwise, tip necrosis may occur. Downward incision follows the anterior border of the trapezius muscle.
- Recommendation: use modified Schobinger approach, but discuss MacFee incision in irradiated patients and patients with a short neck.

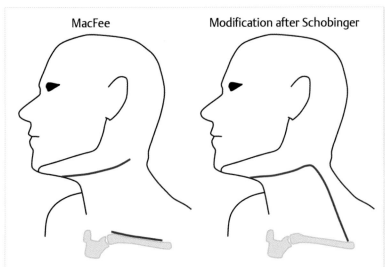

MacFee   Modification after Schobinger

Fig. 2.27 MacFee incision and modified Schobinger approach to levels IV and V.

2.3.2 Relevant Anatomy for Level V Dissection

- The leading landmark for dissection of level V is the greater auricular nerve.

- The most severe malpractice that can occur during dissection of level V is injury of the SAN.
- Location of the SAN: 1 cm cranial of the point where the greater auricular nerve fades away behind the posterior border of the SCM muscle (Fig. 2.28).

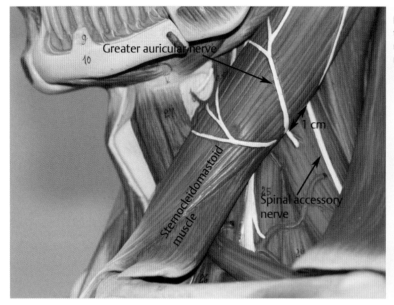

Fig. 2.28 Anatomy of the lateral posterior triangle (landmarks: SCM muscle, trapezius muscle, clavicle), shown on anatomic torso model (SOMSO, Coburg, Germany).

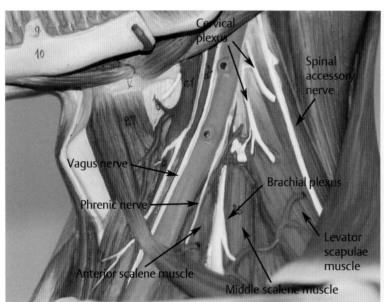

Fig. 2.29 Anatomy of the lateral posterior triangle after removal of the SCM muscle, shown on anatomic torso model (SOMSO).

2.3.3 Technique of Posterior Neck Dissection (MacFee Approach)

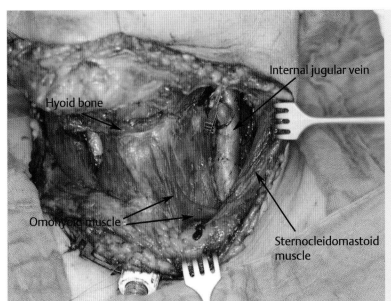

Fig. 2.30 View following neck dissection of levels I to III, anterior view.

Internal jugular vein

Hyoid bone

Omohyoid muscle

Sternocleidomastoid muscle

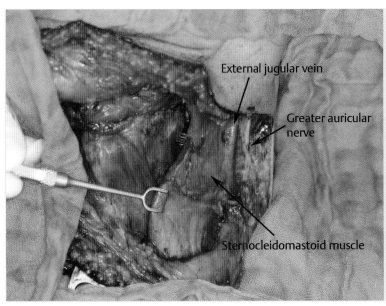

Fig. 2.31 Visualization of the external jugular vein and the greater auricular nerve on the SCM muscle surface, anterolateral view.

External jugular vein

Greater auricular nerve

Sternocleidomastoid muscle

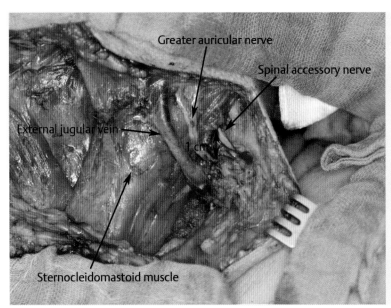

Fig. 2.32 Preparation of the posterior border of the SCM muscle and exposure of the point at which the greater auricular nerve disappears behind the SCM muscle. Following the posterior border from that point 1 cm superiorly to the mastoid, the SAN becomes visible.

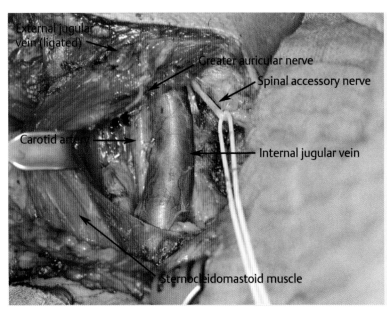

Fig. 2.33 Dissection of the SAN in distal direction, resulting in visualization of the anterior border of the trapezius muscle. Dissection of the fat and lymphoid tissue located caudally and anteriorly of the SAN from the deep cervical fascia. Do not cut the deep cervical fascia.

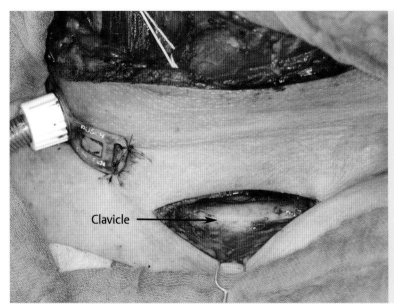

Fig. 2.34 In short necks: second incision at the level of the clavicle (MacFee incision). Subcutaneous dissection in cranial direction to preserve a skin bridge.

Clavicle

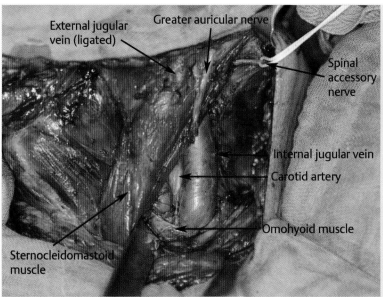

Fig. 2.35 Retraction of the SCM muscle in an anterior direction and the skin bridge in a caudal direction. Preparation of the IJV in a caudal direction and visualization of the intermediate tendon of the omohyoid muscle crossing the IJV. Exposure of the inferior part of the omohyoid muscle to the point at which it is crossed by the clavicle.

External jugular vein (ligated)

Greater auricular nerve

Spinal accessory nerve

Internal jugular vein

Carotid artery

Omohyoid muscle

Sternocleidomastoid muscle

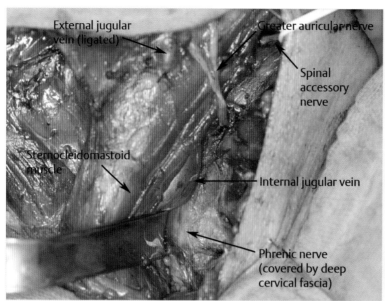

Fig. 2.36 Removal of the fatty and lymphoid tissue package from an anterior (IJV) to posterior (trapezius muscle) direction; avoid cutting the deep cervical fascia. Ligation of the transverse cervical artery and its comitant vein, which runs through the above-mentioned package. Avoid subclavicular preparation which may cause thoracic duct injury on the left side. Avoid injury of the phrenic nerve running anteriorly of the anterior scalene muscle and of the brachial plexus passing between the anterior and middle scalenes.

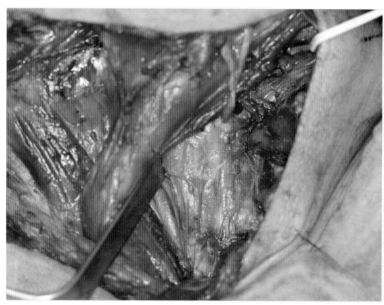

Fig. 2.37 Status after removal of levels IV and V.

2.3.4 Alternative Approaches for Levels I to V

Modified Schobinger Approach

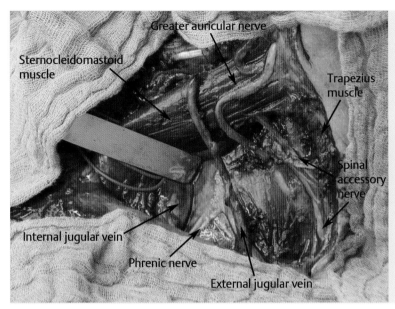

Fig. 2.38 Overview after posterior neck dissection via modified Schobinger approach.

Greater auricular nerve

Sternocleidomastoid muscle

Trapezius muscle

Spinal accessory nerve

Internal jugular vein

Phrenic nerve

External jugular vein

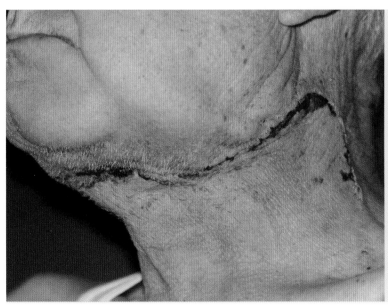

Fig. 2.39 Results on the 12th postoperative day after removal of sutures; the vertical incision of the cranioposterior tip of the skin flap has to be at least 90° to avoid tip necrosis.

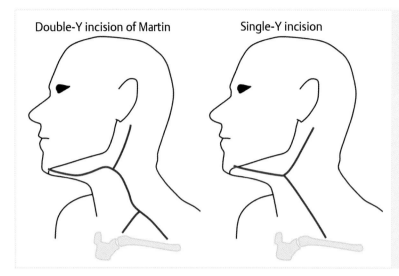

Double-Y incision of Martin

Single-Y incision

Fig. 2.40 Double-Y incision of Martin: good overview, but problematic blood perfusion at the crossing points. Single-Y incision: difficult overview on levels IV and V.

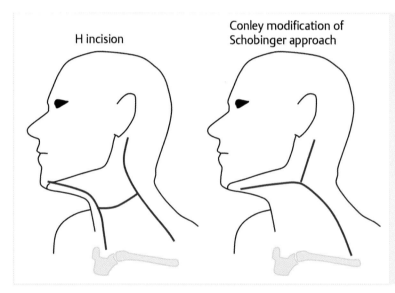

H incision

Conley modification of Schobinger approach

Fig. 2.41 H incision: excellent overview on levels I to V. Conley modification of Schobinger approach: protects the carotid artery.

Recommended Reading

Bocca E, Pignataro O. A conservation technique in radical neck dissection. Ann Otol Rhinol Laryngol 1967; 76: 975–987

Bocca E, Pignataro O, Sasaki CT. Functional neck dissection. A description of operative technique. Arch Otolaryngol 1980; 106: 524–527

Bocca E, Pignataro O, Oldini C, Cappa C. Functional neck dissection: an evaluation and review of 843 cases. Laryngoscope 1984; 94: 942–945

Crile GW. On the surgical treatment of cancer of the head and neck. With a summary of one hundred and twenty-one operations performed upon one hundred and five patients. Trans South Surg Gynecol Assoc. 1905; 18: 108–127

Crile G. Excision of cancer of the head and neck. With special reference to the plan of dissection based on one hundred and thirty-two operations. JAMA 1906; 47: 1780–1786

Jawdynski F. Przypadek raka pierwotnego szyi. t.z. raka skrzelowego Volkmann'a. Wycieecie nowotworu wraz z rezekcyjea teetnicy szyjowej wspólnej i zyly szyjowej wewneetrznej. Wyzdrowienie. Gaz Lek. 1888; 8: 530–537

MacFee WF. Transverse incisions for neck dissection. Ann Surg 1960; 151: 279–284

Robbins KT, Medina JE, Wolfe GT, Levine PA, Sessions RB, Pruet CW. Standardizing neck dissection terminology. Official report of the Academy's Committee for Head and Neck Surgery and Oncology. Arch Otolaryngol Head Neck Surg. 1991; 117: 601–5

Schobinger R. The use of a long anterior skin flap in radical neck resections. Ann Surg 1957; 146: 221–223

Suárez O. Le probleme chirurgical du cancer du larynx. Ann Otolaryngol. 1962; 79: 22–34

Suárez O. El problema de las metastasis linfaticas y alejadas del cancer de laringe e hipofaringe. Rev Otorrinolaringol 1963; 23: 83–99

Suen JY, Goepfert H. Standardization of neck dissection nomenclature. Head Neck Surg 1987; 10: 75–77

Chapter 3
Ablative Tumor Surgery

3.1   Access to the Tumor and Tumor
        Resection   34

3.2   Lip-split Mandibulotomy Access   34

3.3   Weber-Fergusson-Dieffenbach
        Approach   41

3.4   Midfacial Degloving   43

3.5   Le Fort I Osteotomy Approach   46

3.6   Tumor Access: Further
        Approaches   47

3.7   Tumor Resection   48

        Recommended Reading   49

3.1 Access to the Tumor and Tumor Resection

3.1.1 Overview and Accessibility

Obtaining clear margins is the single most important factor in ablative tumor surgery. The anatomy of the oral cavity and its neighboring tissues does not provide ideal conditions to approach all types of tumors in their whole circumference. Tumors of the tongue base and the soft palate region and extended neoplasms with infiltration of the skull base, the sinus region, or the pterygopalatine fossa may not be removed completely via an intraoral approach. Alternative procedures are recommended in the following section.

3.1.2 Alternative Approaches and Indications

Lip-split Mandibulotomy Access

Neoplasms of the pterygomandibular region, the tongue base, and the oropharynx.

Weber-Fergusson-Dieffenbach Approach

Extended neoplasms of the maxilla, the maxillary sinus, and the adjacent anatomical structures.

Midfacial Degloving

Extended neoplasms of the maxilla with infiltration into the central midface and nasal cavity.

Le Fort I Osteotomy

Neoplasms of the maxilla including the anterior and middle parts of the maxillary sinus.

3.2 Lip-split Mandibulotomy Access

3.2.1 History

In 1836, the French surgeon Philibert Joseph Roux introduced one of the most important procedures for oral cancer surgery: the division of lip and mandible to gain access to the floor of the mouth and the tongue. Born in 1780 in Auxerre, he not only influenced oncologic surgery, but also cleft surgery. Roux was probably the first to establish a successful technique for soft palate closure. Although Albrecht von Graefe carried out his first soft palate closure in 1816, the technique was successful in only one patient because he cauterized the cleft margins. Roux did not cauterize the margins but performed surgical debridement before suturing and achieved excellent results by using his own technique in 1819.

3.2.2 Modifications

Modifications were suggested regarding the soft tissue incision and the osteotomy line.

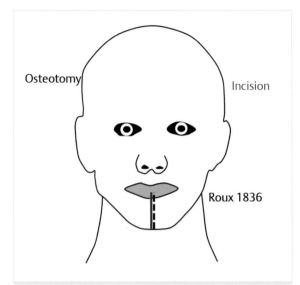

Fig. 3.1 Original incision by Roux, 1836. Roux cut a straight line vertically through the lip midline and the chin.

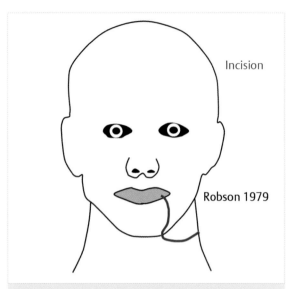

Fig. 3.2 After Robson, 1979. Martin Robson (Chicago) does not start in the lip midline, but medial of the oral commissure, touches the lateral aspect of the chin, and runs downward to the neck incision.

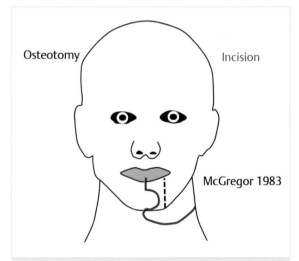

Fig. 3.3 After McGregor, 1983. Ian McGregor (Glasgow) incises the lip midline extending in a vertical fashion toward the chin, then circulating the chin and running downward into the neck incision.

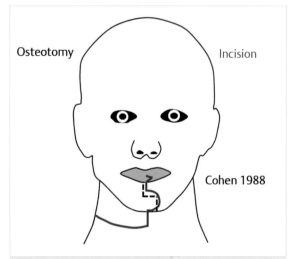

Fig. 3.4 After Cohen, 1988. James Cohen (Minneapolis) suggested the stairstep osteotomy, which allows exact repositioning of the mandibular segments.

3.2.3 Technique

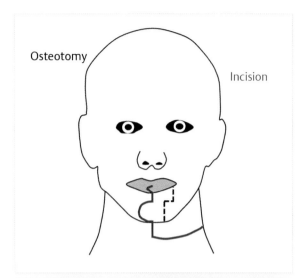

Fig. 3.5 Schematic drawing of skin incisions and stairstep osteotomy line. Note: triangular incision in the lip vermillion for exact repositioning.

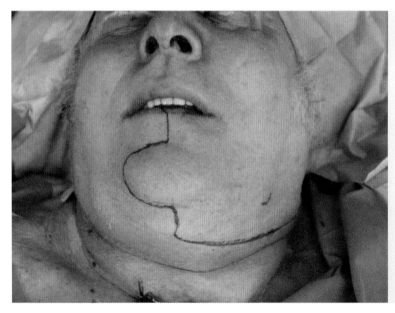

Fig. 3.6 Marking the skin incision.

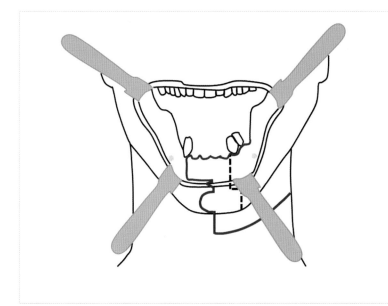

Fig. 3.7 Schematic drawing of intra- and extraoral incision line.

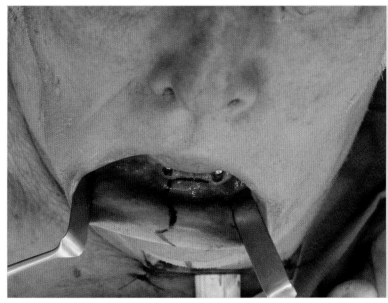

Fig. 3.8 Cut the attached mandibular gingiva paramedially on the contralateral side of the osteotomy to gain more soft tissue coverage for the osteosynthesis material.

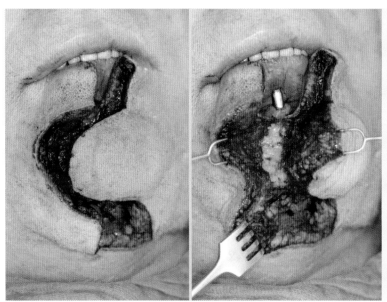

Fig. 3.9 Extraoral and intraoral soft tissue incision, exposure of the mandibula.

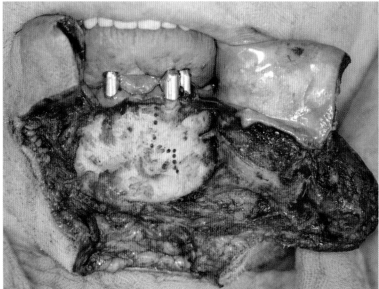

Fig. 3.10 Mark the paramedian stairstep osteotomy line.

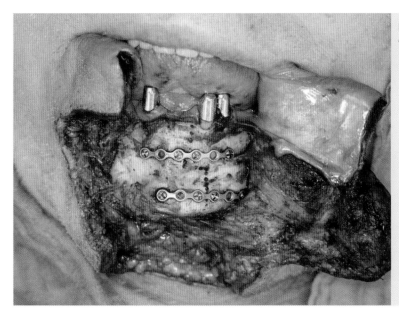

Fig. 3.11 Perform the osteosynthesis before osteotomy, then remove plates and screws.

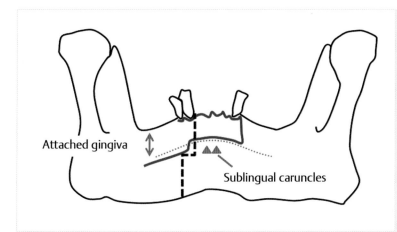

Attached gingiva

Sublingual caruncles

Fig. 3.12 Schematic drawing of the lingual incision. Make the lingual incision on the caudal border of the attached gingiva, save the sublingual caruncles, and extend the incision from the lateral floor of the mouth to the tumor region.

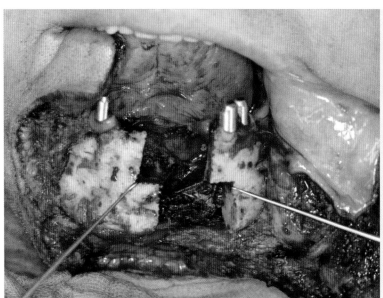

Fig. 3.13 Scrape lingual soft tissue off bone. Protect lingual soft tissue with orbital spatula. Carry out the stairstep osteotomy with a saw.

3.3 Weber-Fergusson-Dieffenbach Approach

3.3.1 History

The history of this approach remains puzzling. After taking many sources into account, Sir William Fergusson (1808–1877), a Scottish surgeon, described an approach to maxillary resection in his book *A System of Practical Surgery* in 1845. Karl Otto Weber, who was born in 1827 in Frankfurt am Main, became head of the surgical department of Heidelberg University in 1865. Some sources attribute the first description of the midfacial approach to his publication from Heidelberg "Vorstellung einer Kranken mit Resection des Unterkiefers" in 1845. With respect to Weber's date of birth, that seems quite illusory. Later, Weber described access to the midface in Pitha and Billroth's surgical handbook, which was published in 1866—one year before he died from diphtheria at the age of 39. Johann Friedrich Dieffenbach's (1792–1847) contribution appears to rely exclusively on the lateral extension to the lower eyelid. A closer look at his contributions to oral cancer surgery can be found in section 4.2.

3.3.2 Technique

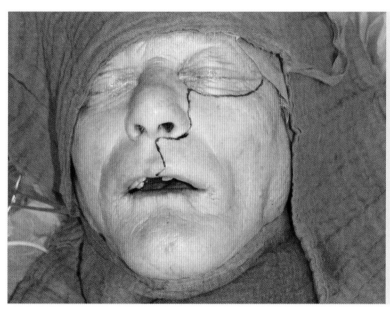

Fig. 3.14 Patient in supine position with entire face prepared and appropriate draping around the surgical area. Start with a zigzag incision of the lip vermillion to the white roll followed by an extraoral skin incision following the ipsilateral philtrum. Then, proceed around the base of the nose and incise along the nasal vestibule to the medial canthus.

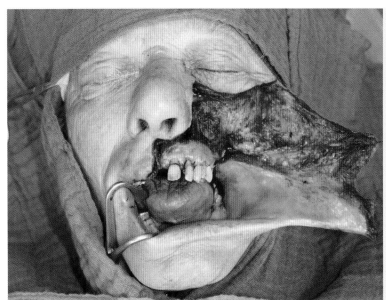

Fig. 3.15 Intraoral incision from the lip vermillion in a vertical direction to the upper mucolabial fold and transverse cut in the mucolabial fold to the maxillary tuberosity. If anterior wall of the maxillary sinus is not affected by the tumor, then use epiperiostal preparation; otherwise, use subcutaneous preparation of the cheek flap. Subciliary incision extraorally through the orbicularis oculi muscle down to the bone extending to the lateral canthus followed by lateral fixation of the cheek flap with sutures.

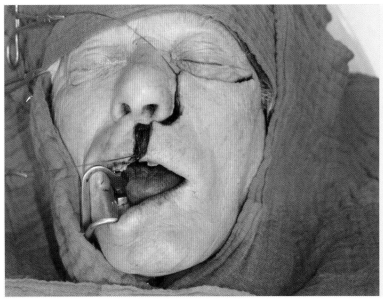

Fig. 3.16 Cheek flap turned back in medial direction.

3.4 Midfacial Degloving

3.4.1 History

1974

John Marquis Converse (1909–1981) established the procedure at the New York University Medical Center. He was born in San Francisco, went to school in Paris, and obtained his medical degree in France. Then, he moved back to the United States to do his residency. His further life as a surgeon was characterized by specializing in craniofacial reconstructive surgery. In 1963, he took over the direction of the Institute of Reconstructive Plastic Surgery at New York University. Interestingly, he was married from 1964 until his death to Veronica Cooper, the widow of film legend Gary Cooper.

3.4.2 Technique

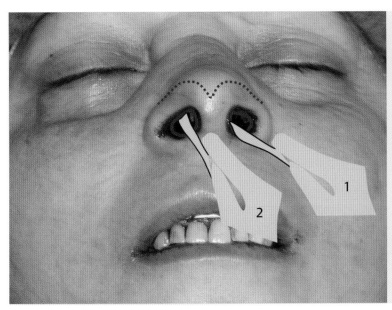

Fig. 3.17 Incision through the nasal mucosa (1) posterior to the greater alar cartilage (2) and anterior of the lateral cartilage (intercartilaginous incision). Similar procedure on the contralateral side. Mandibulomaxillary fixation with trauma splints to retain a correct jaw relationship postoperatively is mandatory.

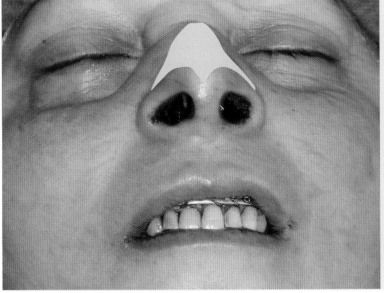

Fig. 3.18 Dissection of the soft tissue overlying the lateral cartilages as far as the nasal bone.

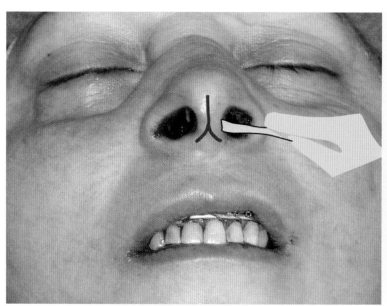

Fig. 3.19 Cut the septal cartilage dorsally and anteriorly.

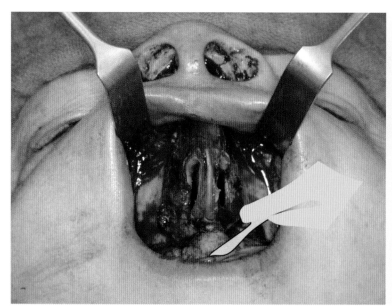

Fig. 3.20 Intraoral incision of the vestibulum.

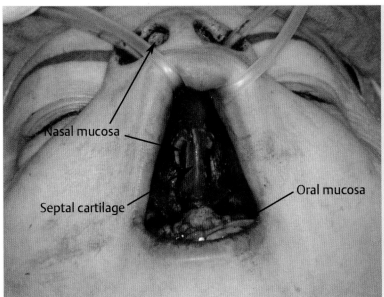

Fig. 3.21 Completed dissection with anatomic landmarks.

Nasal mucosa

Septal cartilage

Oral mucosa

3.5 Le Fort I Osteotomy Approach

3.5.1 History

1859

Bernhard von Langenbeck (1810–1887) succeeded Dieffenbach as head of surgery and ophthalmology at the Charité in Berlin. In 1859, he carried out the pioneer procedure for osteotomy and temporary mobilization of the maxilla in the horizontal plane. After removing a nasopharyngeal polyp via this approach, he observed subsequent healing of the upper jaw in its original position.

1965

As a routine procedure for orthognathic repair, the Le Fort I osteotomy was introduced by Hugo Obwegeser (born in 1920 in Hohenems, Austria) in 1965. From 1964, he was head of Zurich University's department for maxillofacial surgery until his retirement in 1989.

Late 1980s

In the late 1980s, nearly 130 years after von Langenbeck's description, the technique was readapted for tumor surgery of the skull base by a group of British maxillofacial and neurosurgeons led by Daniel Archer and David Uttley. American otolaryngologist Judson R. Belmont also described the use of this technique in 1988. In 1990, Clarence T. Sasaki (born in 1941 in Honolulu), at Yale School of Medicine, reported about six patients with tumors of the central skull base who were operated on via Le Fort I osteotomy.

3.5.2 Technique

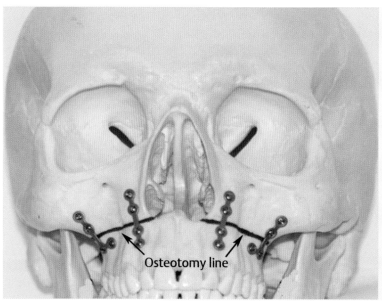

Osteotomy line

Fig. 3.22 Anatomic model of the Le Fort I osteotomy line.

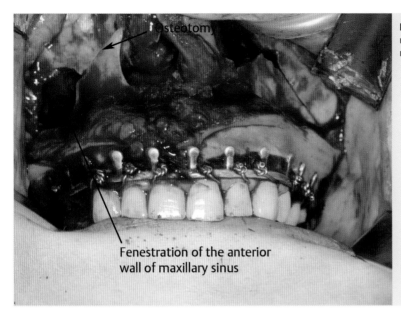

Osteotomy

Fenestration of the anterior
wall of maxillary sinus

Fig. 3.23 Intraoperative view of osteoto-mized maxilla with fenestration of the right maxilla for flap pedicle.

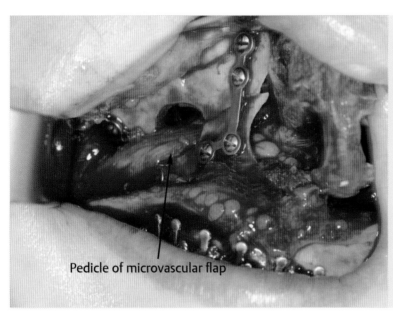

Pedicle of microvascular flap

Fig. 3.24 Osteosynthesis of the maxilla after resection and reconstruction of a palatal malignancy including the central midface. Pedicle of a radial forearm flap running through the maxillary window.

3.6 Tumor Access: Further Approaches

3.6.1 To the Upper Part of the Oral Cavity and the Midface

- Posterior maxillary approach
- Anterolateral corridor approach

3.6.2 To the Lower Part of the Oral Cavity

- "Pull-through" technique/mandibular lingual releasing access
- Visor flap

3.7 Tumor Resection

Obtaining tumor-free margins is the single most important factor in ablative tumor surgery. A margin of 5 mm of uninvolved tissue around the tumor is in accordance with an R0 status in oral squamous cell carcinoma.

3.7.1 Technique

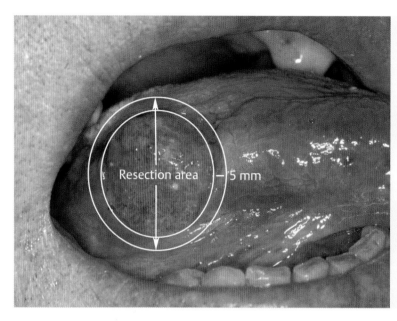

Fig. 3.25 Palpation of the tumor. Excision of the primary tumor by utilization of a 5-mm margin around the visible and palpable tumor in the transverse and vertical dimensions.

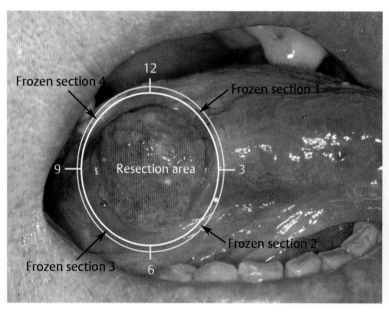

Fig. 3.26 Clockwise mapping of the tumor in the horizontal dimension. Excision of four random tissue pieces of 2-mm width for frozen sectioning.

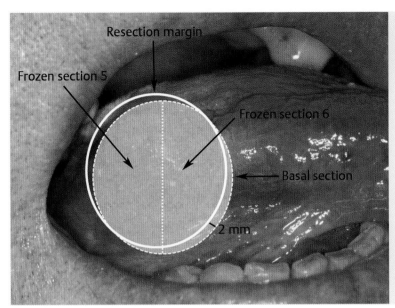

Fig. 3.27 Excision of another two semilunar basal random tissue pieces of 2-mm thickness.

Recommended Reading

Archer DJ, Young S, Uttley D. Basilar aneurysms: a new transclival approach via maxillotomy. J Neurosurg 1987; 67: 54–58

Belmont JR. The Le Fort I osteotomy approach for nasopharyngeal and nasal fossa tumors. Arch Otolaryngol Head Neck Surg 1988; 114: 751–754

Butlin HT. Diseases of the tongue. London: Cassell; 1885: 331

Casson PR, Bonanno PC, Converse JM. The midface degloving procedure. Plast Reconstr Surg 1974; 53: 102–103

Cohen JI, Marentette LJ, Maisel RH. The mandibular swing stabilization of the midline mandibular osteotomy. Laryngoscope 1988; 98: 1139–1142

Fergusson W. A system of practical surgery. Part IV. Chapter 10. Operations on the jaw. 2nd ed. Philadelphia: Lea and Blanchard; 1845:515–532

Fernandes R, Ord R. Access surgery for oral cancer. Oral Maxillofac Surg Clin North Am 2006; 18: 565–571

McGregor IA, MacDonald DG. Mandibular osteotomy in the surgical approach to the oral cavity. Head Neck Surg 1983; 5: 457–462

Obwegeser H. Surgery of the maxilla for the correction of prognathism. SSO Schweiz Monatsschr Zahnheilkd. 1965; 75: 365-74. German.

Robson MC. An easy access incision for the removal of some intraoral malignant tumors. Plast Reconstr Surg 1979; 64: 834–835

Sasaki CT, Lowlicht RA, Astrachan DI, Friedman CD, Goodwin WJ, Morales M. Le Fort I osteotomy approach to the skull base. Laryngoscope 1990; 100: 1073–1076

Uttley D, Moore A, Archer DJ. Surgical management of midline skull-base tumors: a new approach. J Neurosurg 1989; 71: 705–710

von Langenbeck B. Beiträge zur Osteoplastik: Die Osteoplastische Resektion des Oberkiefers. In: A Goschen, ed. Deutsche Klinik. Berlin: Reimer; 1859

Weber KO. Die Krankheit des Gesichts. In: Pitha V, Billroth T, eds. Handbuch der allgemeinen und speziellen Chirurgie. Stuttgart: Verlag Ferdinand Enke; 1866–1873:65–402

Weber O. Vorstellung einer Kranken mit Resection des Unterkiefers. Verhandlungen des naturhist-med Vereins z Heidelberg. 1845;4:80–82

Chapter 4
Reconstructive Surgery

4.1	Considerations on Reconstructive Procedures	52
4.2	Suggestions for Reconstructive Algorithms	52
4.3	Nasolabial Flap	54
4.4	Deltopectoral Flap	60
4.5	Microvascular Anastomosis	66
4.6	Radial Forearm Flap	70
4.7	Anterolateral Thigh Flap/ Myocutaneous Vastus Lateralis Flap	75
4.8	Osseocutaneous Fibula Flap	85
4.9	Considerable Alternatives in Reconstruction	96
4.10	Principles of Complex Reconstruction Planning	97
	Recommended Reading	118

4.1 Considerations on Reconstructive Procedures

Ablative tumor surgery in the oral cavity results in loss of tissue and function. Except for some minor cases, which can be closed primarily, reconstruction is a pivotal aspect of oral cancer surgery. To regain sufficient speech, deglutition, and mastication, transfer of suitable tissue into the oral cavity is unavoidable. The reconstructive ladder is a valuable tool for the proper planning of intraoral restoration. With a significant number of patients suffering from serious comorbidities, the surgeon has to consider the reconstructive procedure carefully. Reconstructive procedures themselves are accompanied by significant donor site morbidity. Thus, one step down the reconstructive ladder may yield far better overall results in elderly and comorbid patients.

4.2 Suggestions for Reconstructive Algorithms

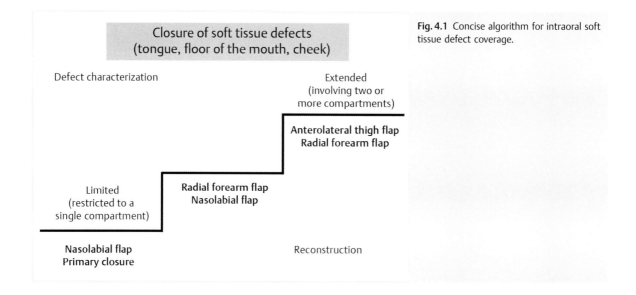

Closure of soft tissue defects (tongue, floor of the mouth, cheek)

Defect characterization

Extended (involving two or more compartments)

**Anterolateral thigh flap
Radial forearm flap**

Limited (restricted to a single compartment)

**Radial forearm flap
Nasolabial flap**

**Nasolabial flap
Primary closure**

Reconstruction

Fig. 4.1 Concise algorithm for intraoral soft tissue defect coverage.

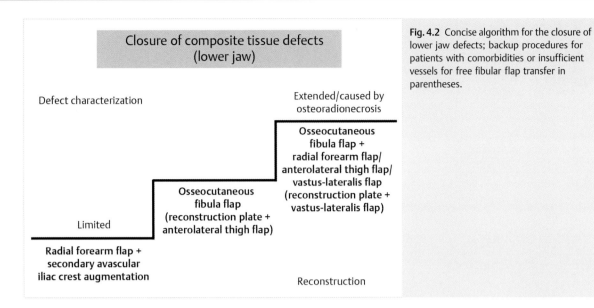

Fig. 4.2 Concise algorithm for the closure of lower jaw defects; backup procedures for patients with comorbidities or insufficient vessels for free fibular flap transfer in parentheses.

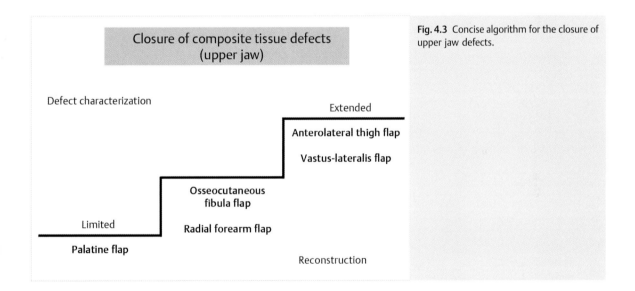

Fig. 4.3 Concise algorithm for the closure of upper jaw defects.

4.3 Nasolabial Flap

4.3.1 History

700/600 BC

Sushruta, an ancient Indian surgeon, described more than 300 operative procedures. His work not only included the famous "Indian forehead flap" to reconstruct the nose, but also the nasolabial flap.

1830

Johann Friedrich Dieffenbach was born in 1792 in Königsberg/East Prussia and was the head of the surgical department at the Charité in Berlin by the time he died in 1847. He described the use of the superiorly based nasolabial flap to reconstruct the nasal alae.

1864

Bernhard von Langenbeck (1810–1887) succeeded Dieffenbach as director of the Clinical Institute for Surgery and Ophthalmology at the Charité in Berlin and remained there until 1882. Langenbeck used the nasolabial flap to reconstruct the nose.

1918

Johannes F. S. Esser (1877–1946) was one of the first "global players" in surgery. After undertaking his medical and surgical education, mainly in the Netherlands, August Bier (1861–1949), the pioneer in anesthesiology, strongly advised Esser to practice in Berlin. During his time in Berlin, he described the nasolabial flap for intraoral reconstruction, in particular the closure of palatal fistulae.

4.3.2 Flap Anatomy

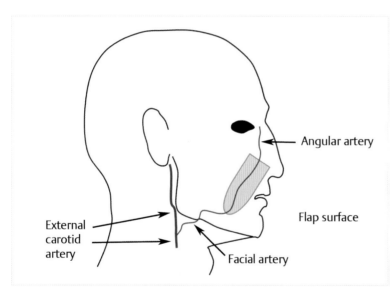

Fig. 4.4 As an axial pattern flap (except the tip), the nasolabial flap receives its blood supply from the facial and angular artery.

Angular artery

Flap surface

External carotid artery

Facial artery

4.3.3 Indications

- Medically compromised patients with localized oral carcinomas. They benefit from reduced operation time (nasolabial flap reconstruction) more than from time-consuming microvascular reconstructions.
- Elderly patients with increased skin laxity in the naso-labial region.
- More appropriate for women because of their hairless nasolabial skin.

- Reconstructions of the anterior region of the oral cavity.

4.3.4 Variations

- Superiorly based for maxillary reconstructions
- Inferiorly based for mandibular and tongue/floor of the mouth reconstructions

4.3.5 Technique

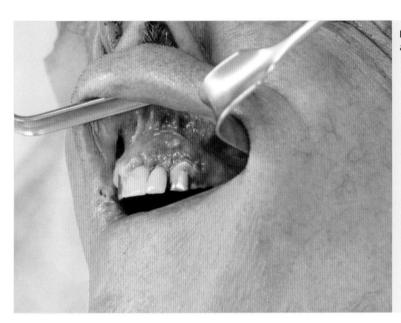

Fig. 4.5 Squamous cell carcinoma of the alveolar ridge of the maxilla.

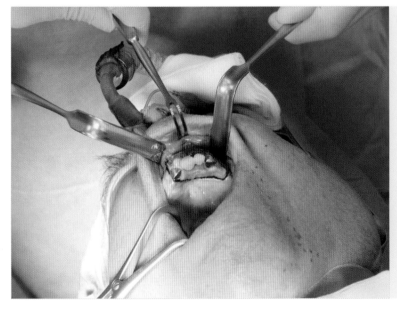

Fig. 4.6 Marking the resection margins.

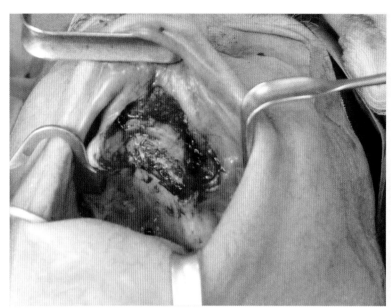

Fig. 4.7 Status after resection of the alveolar ridge carcinoma.

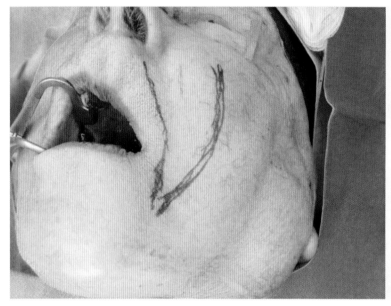

Fig. 4.8 Skin incision outline of the superiorly based nasolabial flap.

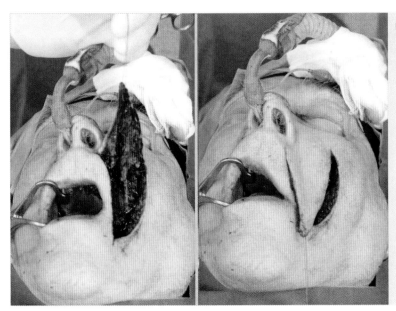

Fig. 4.9 Nasolabial flap harvested.

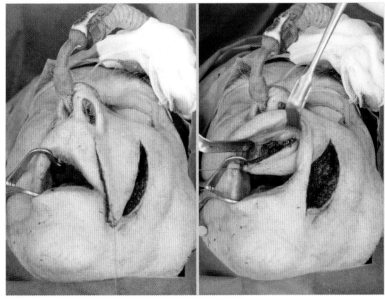

Fig. 4.10 Tunneling through the cheek: "pull through" of the flap and inset into the recipient site.

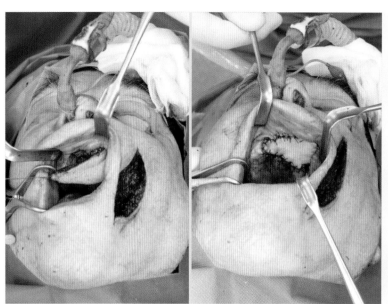

Fig. 4.11 Coverage of the defect by the nasolabial flap and de-epithelization of the tunneled portion of the flap.

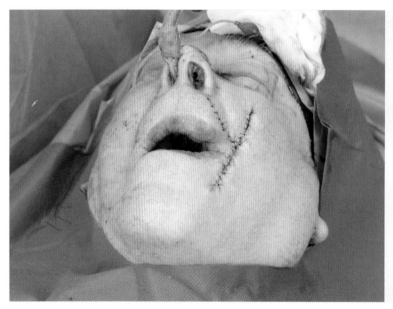

Fig. 4.12 Primary closure of the donor site.

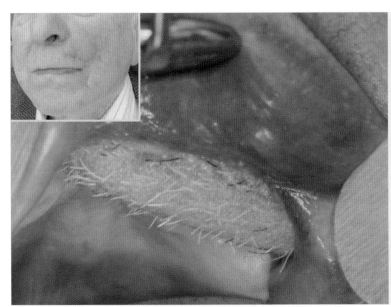

Fig. 4.13 Extraoral and intraoral views of donor and recipient sites 6 months postoperatively. Disadvantage: intraoral reconstruction with hirsute tissue.

4.4 Deltopectoral Flap

4.4.1 History

1917

On November 12, 1917, J.L. Aymard from the Queen Mary's Hospital in Sidcup, United Kingdom, performed a deltopectoral flap operation to reconstruct the nose. The flap did not gain wide acceptance at the time.

1965

Vahram Bakamjian, born 1918 as member of the Armenian minority in Aleppo (Syria), attended the American University of Beirut. After going to the United States in 1951, he did an ear-nose-throat and, later, a plastic surgery residency. From 1956, he worked as a head and neck surgeon in Buffalo where he reintroduced and popularized the "Bakamjian flap" for reconstructive surgery of the head and neck region. He died in 2010 at the age of 92.

4.4.2 Flap Design and Anatomy

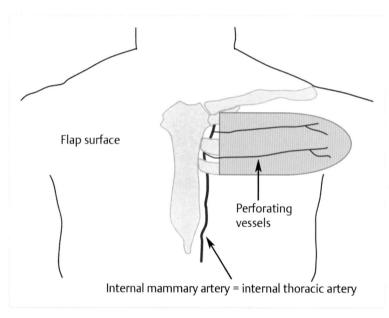

Fig. 4.14 As an axial pattern flap, the deltopectoral flap receives its blood supply from the perforating vessels of the internal mammary artery. If the flap is extended beyond the deltopectoral groove, the tip is a random pattern flap.

Flap surface

Perforating vessels

Internal mammary artery = internal thoracic artery

4.4.3 Indication

"Backup flap" for wound dehiscences after free flap reconstructions, mainly for wound healing disturbances of the irradiated neck.

4.4.4 Technique

First Stage Procedure

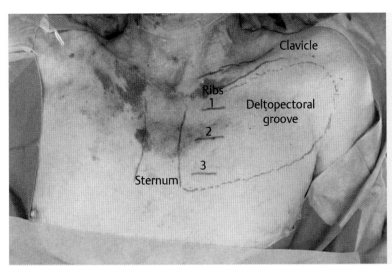

Fig. 4.15 Palpation and marking the landmarks: clavicle, sternum, and ribs 1 to 3. Marking the superior, the inferior, and the lateral extent of the flap. Lateral extension may include a region 3 cm beyond the deltopectoral groove, if necessary. Note: region beyond the deltopectoral groove lies not in the angiosome of the internal mammary perforators, but is a random pattern flap and remains robust in this region.

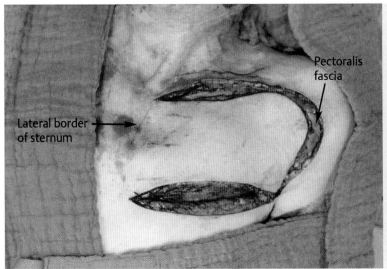

Fig. 4.16 Incision through dermis and subcutaneous fatty tissue onto the pectoralis fascia. Medial incisions should have a distance of 2 cm from the lateral border of the sternum to avoid damaging the perforators.

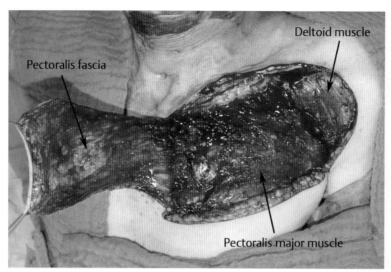

Deltoid muscle

Pectoralis fascia

Pectoralis major muscle

Fig. 4.17 Incision of the pectoralis fascia and integration of the fascia into the flap.

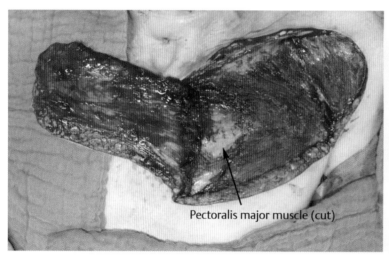

Pectoralis major muscle (cut)

Fig. 4.18 Mobilization of the flap by incising some fibers of the pectoralis major muscle (if necessary), but preserve the region 2 cm lateral of the sternum.

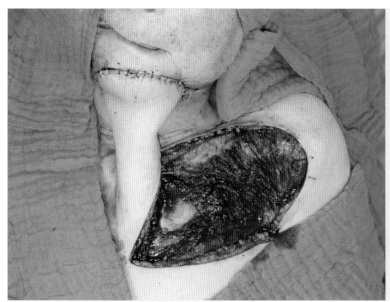

Fig. 4.19 Coverage of the recipient site. Form a tubed pedicle by careful coverage of the tube's inner surface site with artificial dermis. Avoid circumferential closure of the tube pedicle to prevent occlusion of the vessels.

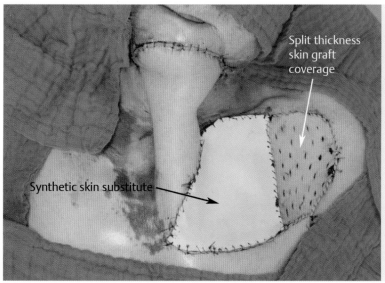

Split thickness skin graft coverage

Synthetic skin substitute

Fig. 4.20 Coverage of the deltopectoral donor site with split thickness skin graft. Temporary coverage of the medially located donor site with a synthetic skin graft.

Second Stage Procedure

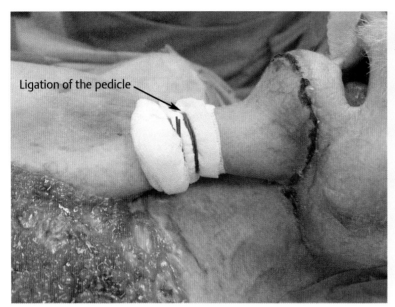

Fig. 4.21 Three weeks after flap harvest: ligation of the flap's pedicle. Controlling flap's autonomization at the recipient site.

Ligation of the pedicle

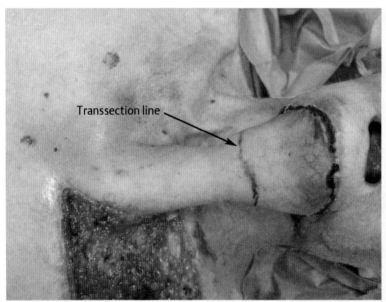

Fig. 4.22 Marking the transsection line.

Transsection line

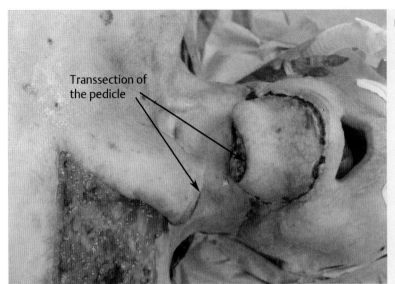

Fig. 4.23 Transsection of the tubed pedicle.

Transsection of
the pedicle

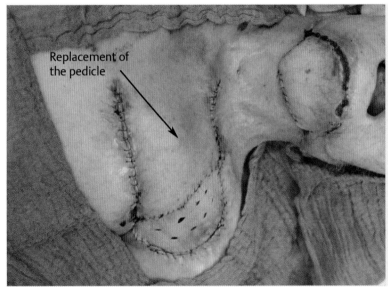

Fig. 4.24 Primary thinning of the transplant at the recipient site and suture. Replacement of the remaining pedicle to the original donor site. Coverage of the remaining distal donor site with split thickness skin graft.

Replacement of
the pedicle

4.5 Microvascular Anastomosis

4.5.1 History

1864

The doctoral thesis of Alexander Jassinowsky was published in German in 1889. His studies were performed in 1864 at the University of Dorpat (today Tartu in Estonia). Jassinowsky had provoked lacerations on the carotid artery of 22 animals and reported successful suturing of the vessels with silk.

1912

Alexis Carrel from Lyon (1873–1944) was awarded the Nobel Prize for pioneering vascular suturing techniques, which formed the basis for transplantation procedures. The medical faculty of Lyon University was named after Carrel until 1994. After coming to terms with its role in implementing eugenics policies during Vichy France, the university deleted his name.

The 1950s

Julius Jacobsen and Ernesto Suarez from Burlington, Vermont, carried out basic work for microvascular anastomosis techniques with a binocular microscope. The research was published in 1960.

1957

On July 30, 1957, Bernard Seidenberg from New York reconstructed the proximal part of the esophagus of a cancer patient with a microvascular pedicled jejunum transplant. This was the first reconstructive procedure using a microvascular anastomosed flap in humans.

1969

Donald McLean and Harry Buncke from Oakland, California, were the first to perform a scalp reconstruction by transferring a microvascular pedicled omentum flap. They published the procedure in 1972.

4.5.2 Technique

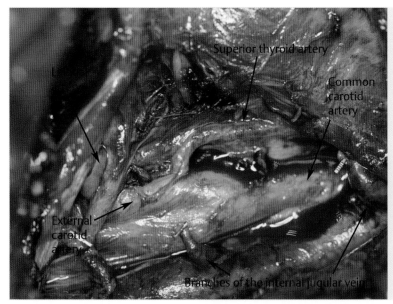

Fig. 4.25 Preparation of suitable recipient vessels as superior thyroid artery or lingual artery on the one hand and direct branches of the internal jugular vein on the other hand.

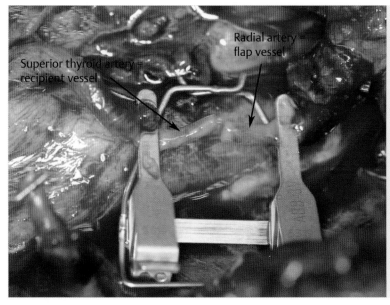

Fig. 4.26 Initial trimming of the adventitia of recipient and donor artery. Approximation of recipient and donor vessel by applying the double clamp.

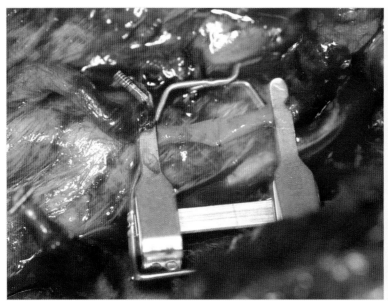

Fig. 4.27 End-to-end triangulation technique: second suture is placed 120° from the first. Sutures are fixed on the opponent edges of the approximator clamp to keep vessel walls under tension and to avoid adhesion of front and back walls (especially in venous anastomosis).

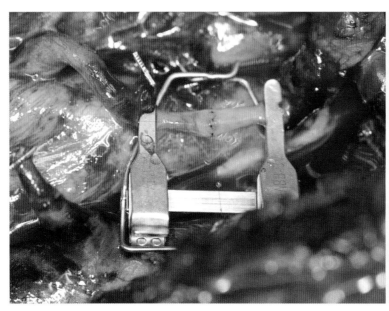

Fig. 4.28 Suturing of front wall is completed; take care of consistent gaps between the sutures.

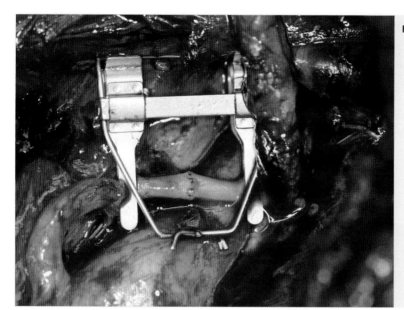

Fig. 4.29 Arterial anastomosis is completed.

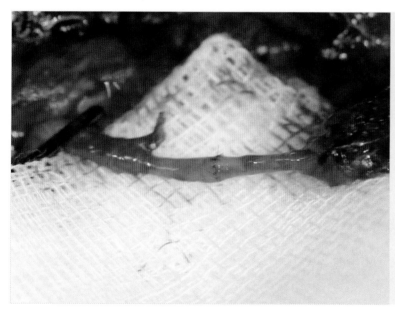

Fig. 4.30 Approximator clamp is removed, but a clamp proximal from the anastomosis is applied. Proximal clamp is not removed until first vein is anastomosed. Confirm no leakage at the anastomosis following release of the clamps.

4.6 Radial Forearm Flap

4.6.1 History

1978

Studies on cadavers investigating the angiosome of the radial forearm flap were first performed by Yang Guo-fan and Gao Yuzhi at the military hospital of Shenyang, China.

In 1981, they published (in Chinese) an initial description of a case study of 56 patients.

1981

In 1980, Wolfgang Mühlbauer from Munich, Klinikum rechts der Isar, traveled together with a German delegation to China and introduced the flap technique to the Western world. The Mühlbauer, Biemer, and Stock working group included the radius to the flap and used the osseocutaneous transplant for thumb reconstruction.

1983

David Soutar and his team from Glasgow described the use of the radial forearm flap for reconstructions of the oral cavity.

4.6.2 Indication

The "workhorse" flap: the universal flap for intraoral reconstruction.

4.6.3 Preliminary Examinations and Considerations

Allen Test

The procedure is named after Edgar Van Nuys Allen (1900–1961), a cardiovascular specialist from the Mayo Clinic in Rochester, Minnesota. The test examines the vascular function of the hand's arteries and perfusion of the vascular palmar arch. In order to detect disturbances in blood circulation and, in consequence, possible postoperative perfusion insufficiencies, both arteries are first occluded by manual compression. The patient is then asked to repeatedly open and close the hand, so the blood is pumped out. Compression of the artery that is to be sacrificed as a future flap pedicle (in this case, the radial artery) is continued, while pressure on the other artery (ulnar artery) is released. It is possible to raise a radial forearm flap without further considerations, if the hand is equally reperfused with blood within 5 seconds.

Handedness

The radial forearm flap should always be raised from the nondominant hand.

4.6.4 Technique

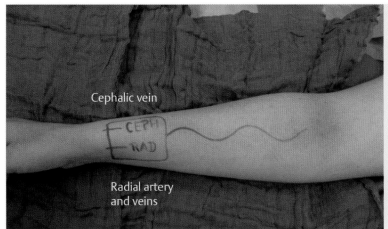

Fig. 4.31 Marking and preparation. Radial orientation: if the cephalic vein is to be included for venous drainage, the marking should be located beyond the brachioradialis muscle. Location of the distal border 1 cm proximal of the most proximal skin crease, when the hand is bent in the volar direction. Define the ulnar border, which can be extended beyond the flexor carpi ulnaris muscle according to the size needed. Define the proximal border by size of the flap, considering the above-mentioned specifications. Mark the radial vessels between the flexor carpi radialis and brachioradialis muscle.

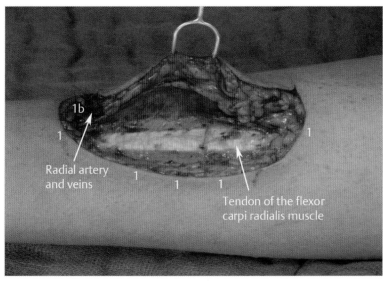

Fig. 4.32 Start the incision from the ulnar part of the flap distally through the skin and the subcutaneous tissue (1). Define the depth by the forearm fascia, which is integrated in the flap. If a large flap is required, expose the tendon of the flexor carpi ulnaris muscle, keeping the paratenon intact. Continue the ulnar-sided flap preparation beyond the tendons of the flexor digitorum and the palmaris longus muscles until reaching the flexor carpi radialis muscle. Localize the radial vessels (pedicle) at the distal end of the flap. The pedicle is running between the flexor carpi radialis and brachioradialis muscle. Ligate the pedicle containing the radial artery and its two comitant veins (1b).

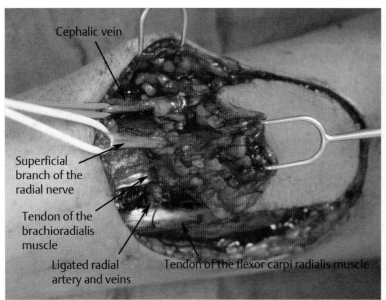

Cephalic vein

Superficial branch of the radial nerve

Tendon of the brachioradialis muscle

Ligated radial artery and veins

Tendon of the flexor carpi radialis muscle

Fig. 4.33 Dissect in radial direction, in order to locate and preserve the superficial branch of the radial nerve, which runs above the tendon of the brachioradialis muscle. Divide the superficial radial nerve in ulnar and radial sections, where the ulnar branch is thinner than the radial branch. Locate and ligate the cephalic vein in the subcutaneous tissue at the radial border of the flap.

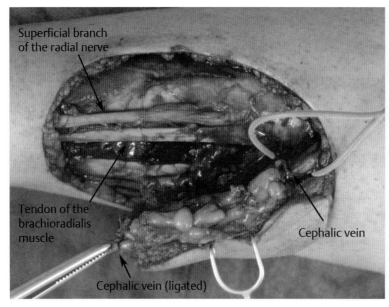

Superficial branch of the radial nerve

Tendon of the brachioradialis muscle

Cephalic vein (ligated)

Cephalic vein

Fig. 4.34 Preparation of the radial border of the flap. Note the course of the cephalic vein: ligation of an anatomic constant radial branch of the cephalic vein, located approximately 3 cm proximal of the distal border. Separate the superficial branch of the radial nerve from the flap tissue. Continue the flap preparation from the distal to the proximal border of the skin island. Locate the vascular pedicle between the flexor carpi radialis and brachioradialis muscles. Carefully dissect the cephalic vein from the brachioradialis tendon, finishing the preparation at the proximal border of the skin island by dissecting cutis and subcutaneous tissue.

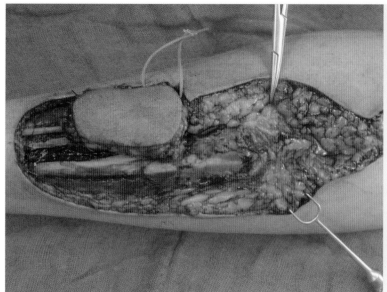

Fig. 4.35 Wave-like incision of the skin and subcutaneous tissue from the middle part of the proximal flap border to the antecubital fossa, until the fascia of the flexor carpi radialis muscle is reached. Identify the cephalic vein at the proximal flap border (blue vessel loop). Dissect the flap while protecting the cephalic vein and the radial pedicle.

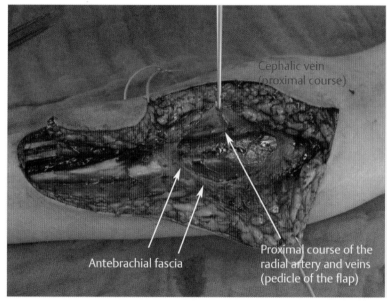

Fig. 4.36 Prepare the cephalic vein from the subcutaneous tissue located radial from the wave-like incision and open the antebrachial fascia at the bottom. Dissect the radial pedicle above the flexor pollicis longus muscle, while small branches to the deep muscles and radial bone are cauterized or clipped. Cut the comitant veins and the cephalic vein at the proximal end of the incision. Evaluate the venous drainage of each single vein. Dissect the radial artery in proximal direction.

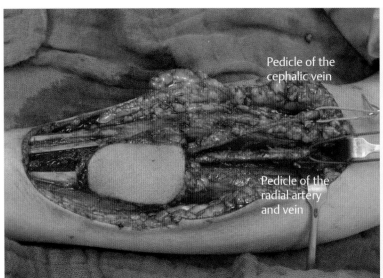

Fig. 4.37 Flap harvest is completed.

4.7 Anterolateral Thigh Flap/ Myocutaneous Vastus Lateralis Flap

4.7.1 History

1984

Song and coworkers described the anterolateral thigh as an additional free flap donor site.

1992

Wolff and coworkers reconstructed the oral cavity by flaps from the anterolateral thigh donor site. They used pure muscle flaps or myofascial flaps from the vastus lateralis muscle; these flaps were pedicled on the descending branch of the lateral circumflex femoral artery.

1996

Kimura and Satoh described primary thinning and defatting of the anterolateral thigh flap and hereby found an effective alternative to the radial forearm flap.

2002

Wei and coworkers raised the question, "Have we found an ideal soft tissue flap?" after harvesting 672 flaps from the anterolateral thigh donor site.

4.7.2 Indication

Huge reconstructions, as thinned anterolateral thigh flap alternative for the radial forearm flap.

4.7.3 Preoperative Procedures

Handheld Doppler ultrasound is used to identify the cutaneous perforator. To determine location of the perforator: draw a line between the anatomic landmarks of the anterior superior iliac spine (ASIS) and lateral patella—the perforator can be found halfway between these landmarks in most cases.

4.7.4 Technique

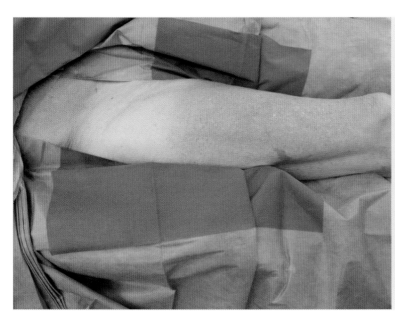

Fig. 4.38 Positioning of the thigh and circumferential skin preparation of lower limb extremity. Anatomic landmarks, ASIS and lateral patella, must be clearly visible and palpable.

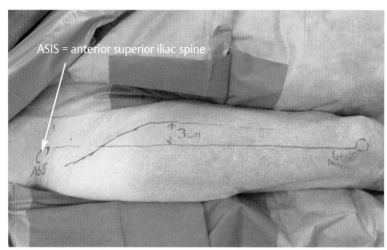

Fig. 4.39 Mark and connect the landmarks of the ASIS and lateral patella by a line. Draw a second line indicating the incision. Incision starts proximally and begins laterally to the interconnecting line. Incision crosses the line and turns to the medial side of the line while keeping a distance of 3 cm. Keeping this distance, the incision runs parallel to the first line in a distal direction.

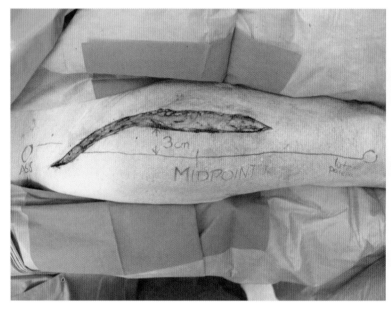

Fig. 4.40 Location of the skin perforator around the midpoint of the connecting line. To avoid accidental laceration of the perforator vessel, the incision must strictly maintain the 3 cm distance from the ASIS/lateral patella line. Incision of skin and subcutaneous tissue down to the fascia of the thigh.

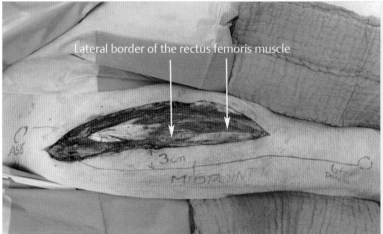

Fig. 4.41 Incision of the rectus femoris muscle fascia. Exposure of the lateral border of the rectus femoris muscle and the intermuscular groove. Demonstration of a septocutaneous perforator running from the intermuscular septum at the undersurface of the rectus femoris muscle in a lateral direction.

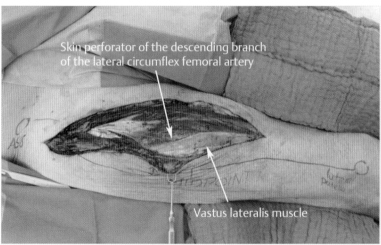

Fig. 4.42 Septocutaneous skin perforator of the descending branch of the lateral circumflex femoral artery seen running on the surface of the vastus lateralis muscle.

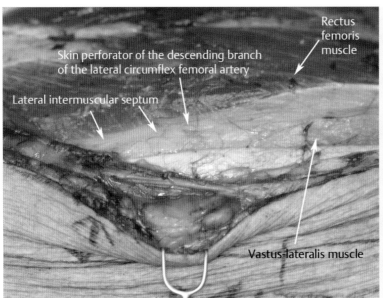

Fig. 4.43 Rectus femoris muscle is retracted slightly medially.

Rectus femoris muscle

Skin perforator of the descending branch of the lateral circumflex femoral artery

Lateral intermuscular septum

Vastus-lateralis muscle

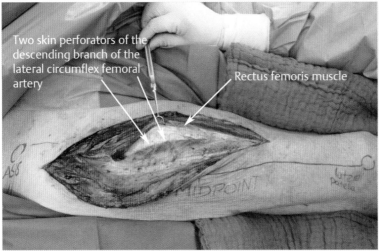

Fig. 4.44 Further retraction of the rectus femoris muscle in a medial direction and identification of a second perforator. Proximally: dissection continues along the muscular groove between the tensor fasciae latae muscle and the rectus femoris muscle. (Tip: blunt dissection with the fingers aids in safe demonstration of the proximal course of the vessels.)

Two skin perforators of the descending branch of the lateral circumflex femoral artery

Rectus femoris muscle

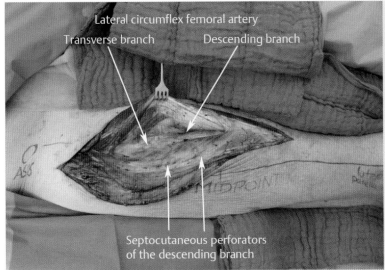

Fig. 4.45 Further retraction of the rectus femoris muscle. The lateral circumflex femoral artery with all its branches becomes visible. The descending branch, with its skin perforators, supplies perfusion for the myocutaneous vastus lateralis/anterolateral thigh flap; the transverse branch or the ascending branch provide perfusion for the myocutaneous tensor fasciae latae flap.

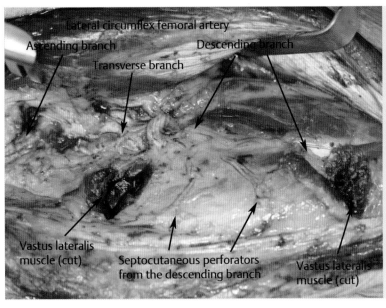

Fig. 4.46 Inclusion of a cuff of vastus lateralis muscle surrounding the perforators into the flap. Therefore, the vastus lateralis muscle is cut in medial-to-lateral direction 2 cm proximal and 2 cm distal from the perforators. This maneuver helps eliminate vascular spasm by avoiding any tension on the perforators.

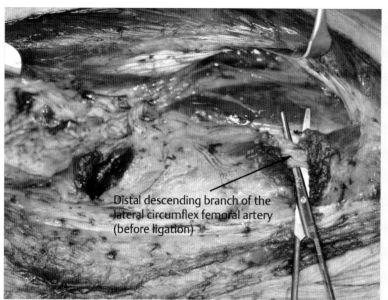

Distal descending branch of the lateral circumflex femoral artery (before ligation)

Fig. 4.47 Ligation of the descending branch 3 cm distal from perforators branching off.

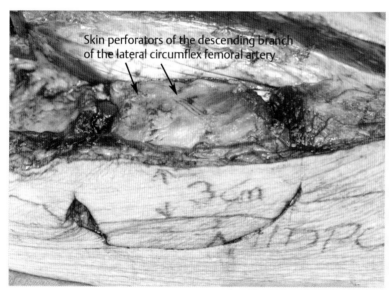

Skin perforators of the descending branch of the lateral circumflex femoral artery

Fig. 4.48 Incision of the skin paddle. Septocutaneous perforators are located in the center of the skin island. Incision of the skin and subcutaneous tissue down to the fascia.

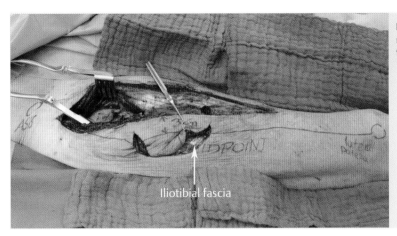

Fig. 4.49 Incision of iliotibial fascia. Perforators must be located in the center of the flap; avoid cutting the fascia too medially.

Iliotibial fascia

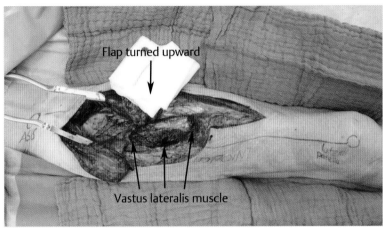

Fig. 4.50 Undermining of the included vastus lateralis muscle part, starting from medial to lateral direction. Separation of the vastus lateralis muscle and inclusion into the flap. Vastus intermedius muscle becomes visible on the base. Flap is turned slightly in a medial direction, the perforators become visible from the undersurface. Cut the iliotibial fascia while keeping a safe distance from the perforators. Fix the fascia to the skin island with resorbable sutures to prevent shearing.

Flap turned upward

Vastus lateralis muscle

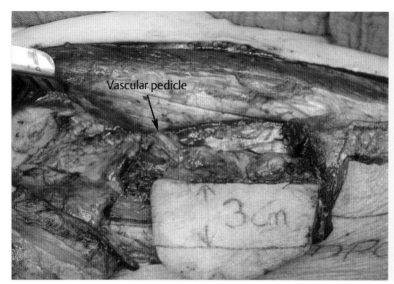

Fig. 4.51 Dissect the vascular pedicle (the descending branch) from distal to proximal direction until reaching its origin from the lateral circumflex femoral vessels.

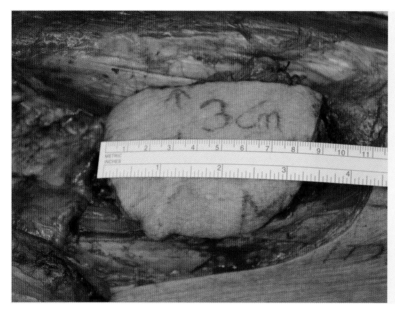

Fig. 4.52 Myocutaneous flap harvest is completed.

4.7.5 Modification of the Procedure by Harvesting an Additional Myocutaneous Tensor Fasciae Latae Flap

History

Foad Nahai, born 1943 in Teheran, and his workgroup from the Emory University Hospital in Atlanta were the first to describe the clinical use of the fascia lata musculocutaneous free flap in 1978.

Indication

When there is a need for two extended skin islands, such as large combined extra- and intraoral defects.

Technique

Initial surgical stages as described until Fig. 4.45.

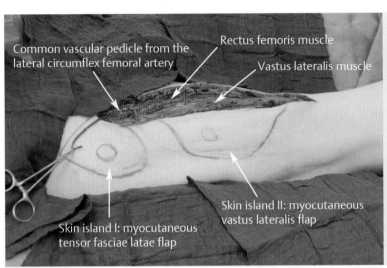

Fig. 4.53 Complete exposure of lateral circumflex femoral artery and its branches between the rectus femoris muscle and vastus lateralis (VL)/tensor fasciae latae (TFL) muscle.

Common vascular pedicle from the lateral circumflex femoral artery

Rectus femoris muscle

Vastus lateralis muscle

Skin island I: myocutaneous tensor fasciae latae flap

Skin island II: myocutaneous vastus lateralis flap

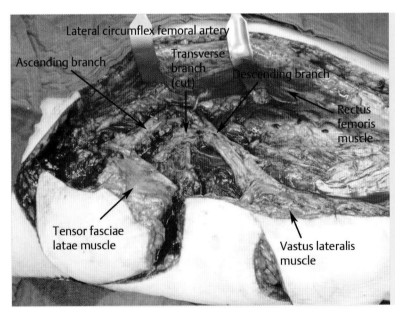

Fig. 4.54 Transverse branch is cut; descending and ascending branches are dissected in distal direction. Skin islands are marked.

Lateral circumflex femoral artery

Ascending branch

Transverse branch (cut)

Descending branch

Rectus femoris muscle

Tensor fasciae latae muscle

Vastus lateralis muscle

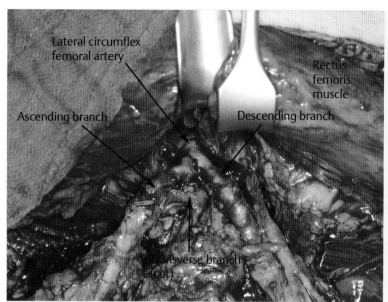

Lateral circumflex
femoral artery

Rectus
femoris
muscle

Ascending branch

Descending branch

Transverse branch
(cut)

Fig. 4.55 Detailed vascular pedicles of myocutaneous TFL and VL flaps.

4.8 Osseocutaneous Fibula Flap

4.8.1 History

1974

On April 7, 1974, Ian Taylor (born 1938 in Melbourne) performed the first vascularized fibula flap transfer to reconstruct parts of the tibia.

1986

Wei et al. popularized the use of the fibula osteoseptocutaneous flap and presented the first 15 clinical cases.

1989

In New York, the first reconstruction of a mandibular defect with a free fibula flap was done by David Hidalgo (born 1952).

1992

Zlotolow and the colleagues of David Hidalgo incorporated secondary osseointegrated dental implants for functional rehabilitation into the neo-mandible constructed from a free fibula flap.

4.8.2 Indication

Composite tissue reconstructions of the lower and upper jaw.

4.8.3 Preoperative Procedures

Clinical Examinations

- Assessment of walking ability (claudication) in patients with peripheral artery occlusive disease
- Palpation of pedal pulses: dorsalis pedis artery and posterior tibial artery
- Use of handheld Doppler probe to mark out the cutaneous perforators (most commonly found at the junction of middle and lower third of the fibula)

Computed Tomography Angiography

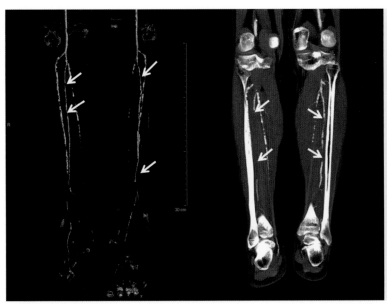

Fig. 4.56 Contraindication for a free fibula flap transfer. Left: anterior view on a three-dimensional (3D) reconstruction showing occlusive disease with insufficient peroneal vessels (*arrows*). Right: posterior view on the interrupted peroneal artery (*arrows*).

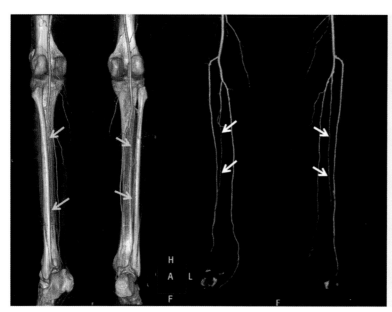

Fig. 4.57 Indication for fibula flap transfer. Left: well-perfused, sufficient peroneal artery, posterior view. Right: sufficient peroneal artery, anterior view on a 3D reconstruction.

4.8.4 Cross-sectional Anatomy

To illustrate fibula flap harvest further, schematic cross-sections to the corresponding clinical stages are included.

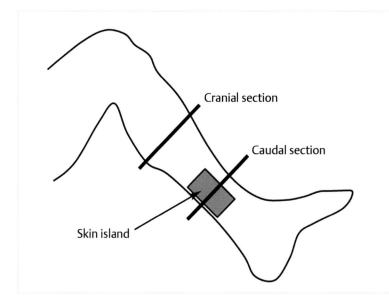

Fig. 4.58 Location of the cranial (see Fig. 4.66a)" and caudal cross-sections of the lower leg.

Cranial section

Caudal section

Skin island

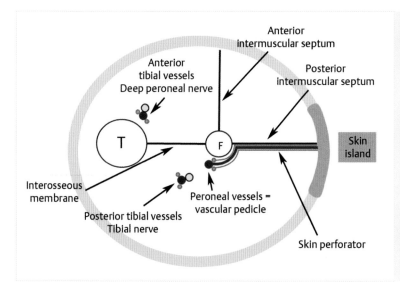

Fig. 4.59 Caudal cross-section of the lower leg: anatomic structures at the level of the skin island. T, tibia; F, fibula.

Anterior intermuscular septum

Anterior tibial vessels
Deep peroneal nerve

Posterior intermuscular septum

T

F

Skin island

Interosseous membrane

Peroneal vessels = vascular pedicle

Posterior tibial vessels
Tibial nerve

Skin perforator

4.8.5 Technique

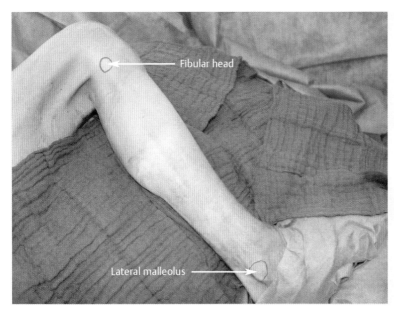

Fig. 4.60 Circumferential preparation of the leg. Fixation of the foot with the knee flexed and moved away from the surgeon. Marking the anatomic landmarks: fibular head and lateral malleolus.

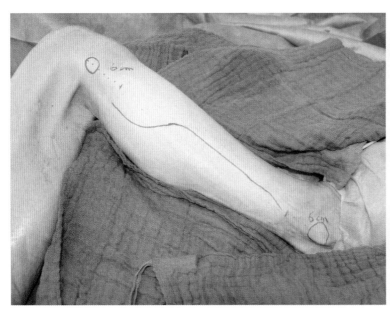

Fig. 4.61 Draw the incision line, starting 6 cm distal of the fibular head so as to preserve the common peroneal nerve, which crosses the fibular neck proximal to this mark. Incision line drawn extending from the lateral to the medial aspect of the underlying posterior intermuscular septum (separating the soleus muscle from the peroneus longus muscle). Incision line stops 6 cm proximal to the lateral malleolus to avoid instability of the ankle.

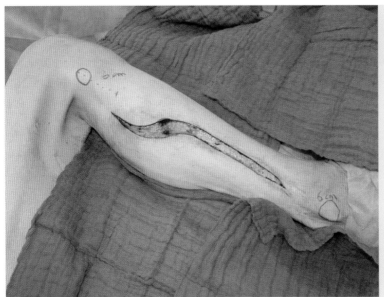

Fig. 4.62 Incision of skin and subcutaneous tissue down to the fascia covering the flexor group of muscles and the peroneus longus muscle.

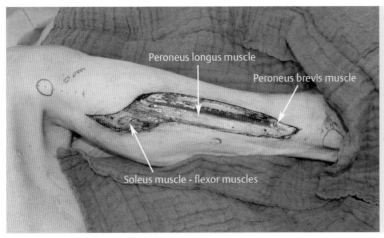

Peroneus longus muscle

Peroneus brevis muscle

Soleus muscle - flexor muscles

Fig. 4.63 Incision of peroneus longus muscle fascia. Separate the peroneus longus muscle, peroneus brevis muscle, and soleus muscle. Blunt and gentle retraction of the skin at the lateral aspect of the peroneus longus muscle; perforator becomes visible next to the Doppler marking.

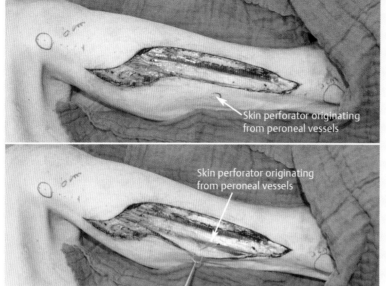

Fig. 4.64 Visualization of the skin perforator in the lateral intermuscular septum.

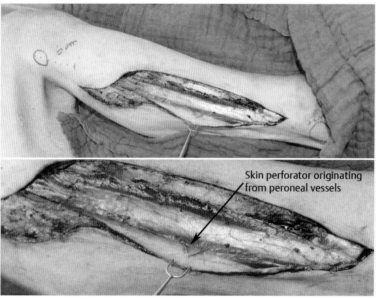

Fig. 4.65 Visualization of the skin perforator in detail.

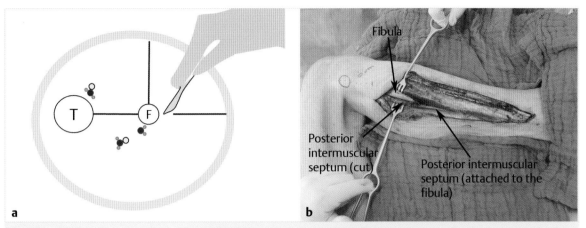

a b

Fig. 4.66 a, b Cranial incision of the lateral intermuscular septum keeping a safe distance to the skin perforator vessels. Cranial detachment of the lateral margin of the fibular bone.

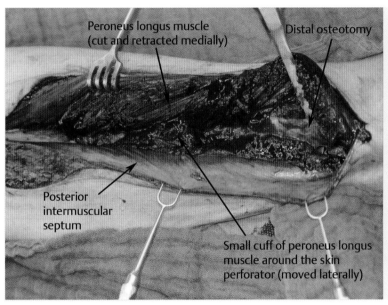

Fig. 4.67 Incision down to the fibula bone from cranial to caudal. Next to the skin perforators, the incision curves medially; in this region, the peroneus longus muscle is incised and a muscle cuff is left laterally to protect the perforator vessel. Carefully and circumferentially dissect the fibular bone with a curved raspatory at the levels of the proximal and distal osteotomy.

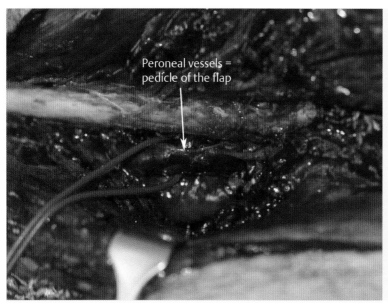

Fig. 4.68 Adjacent to the proximal osteotomy, dissect the tissue located medial to the incised posterior intermuscular septum. Palpate the peroneal vessels. Dissect the peroneal vessels and retract the pedicle in the lateral direction with a vessel loop.

Peroneal vessels = pedicle of the flap

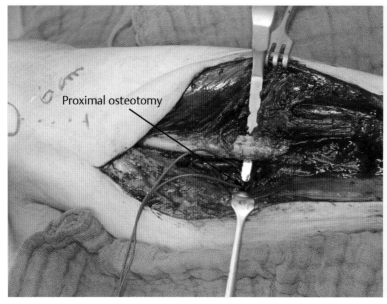

Fig. 4.69 Proximal osteotomy with protection of the pedicle with a raspatory.

Proximal osteotomy

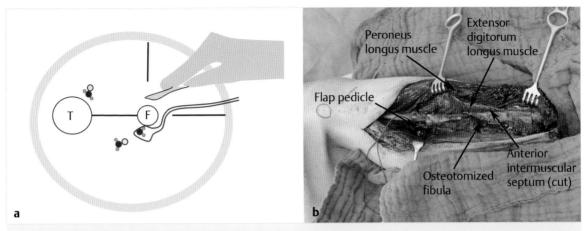

Fig. 4.70 a, b Distal osteotomy with protection of the pedicle with a raspatory. Incision of the anterior intermuscular septum adjacent to the fibula bone; extensor digitorum longus muscle becomes visible.

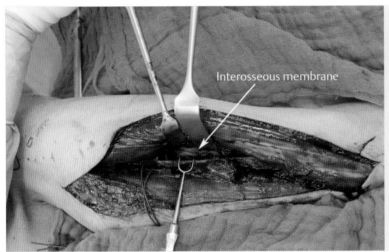

Fig. 4.71 Following retraction of the extensor digitorum longus muscle with hooks, the interosseous membrane becomes visible.

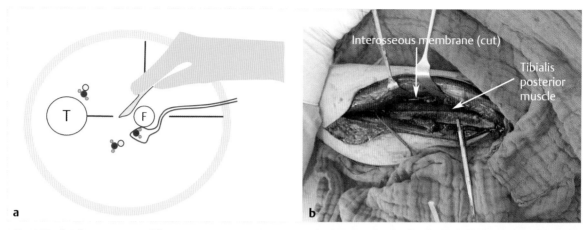

Fig. 4.72 a, b Following incision of the interosseous membrane close to the fibula, the tibialis posterior muscle becomes visible. It is now possible to mobilize the fibula in the lateral direction with a hook.

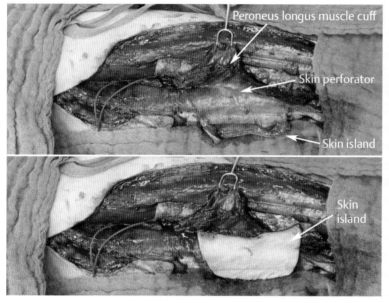

Fig. 4.73 Lateral incision of the skin island while keeping the skin perforator in the center. Try to avoid shearing of the skin island. Careful incision of the posterior intermuscular septum on the underlying soleus muscle. Keep a strict distance of 3 cm to the skin perforators.

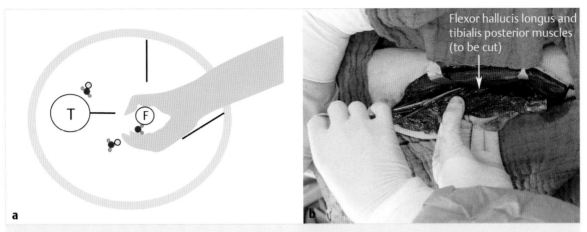

Fig. 4.74a, b Fix the skin island to the periosteum with sutures to avoid shearing. While holding the flap and feeling the pulse of the pedicle between the fingers, the tibialis posterior muscle and the flexor hallucis longus muscle are incised above the fingers.

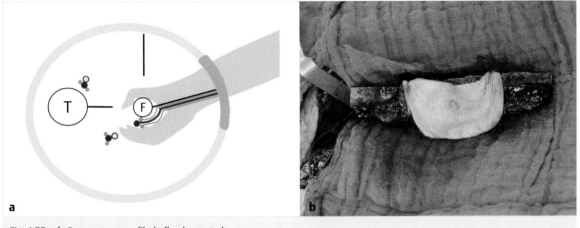

Fig. 4.75a, b Osseocutaneous fibula flap harvested.

4.9 Considerable Alternatives in Reconstruction

4.9.1 Pedicled Flaps

- Temporalis muscle flap
  - Soft tissue reconstruction in the maxillary region
- Platysma flap
  - Soft tissue reconstruction of the floor of the mouth/tongue region
- Pectoralis major flap
  - Extended soft tissue reconstruction for the floor of the mouth/tongue region
  - "Backup flap" for wound dehiscences after free flap reconstructions, mainly for wound healing disturbances of the irradiated neck

- Latissimus dorsi flap
  - Extended soft tissue reconstruction
  - "Backup flap" for wound dehiscences after free flap reconstructions, mainly for wound healing disturbances of the irradiated neck

4.9.2 Free Flaps

- Microvascular reanastomosed latissimus dorsi flap
  - Extended soft tissue reconstruction
- Deep circumflex iliac artery flap (anterior iliac crest bone flap)
  - Bony reconstruction of mandibula or maxilla
- Scapular flap
  - Composite tissue reconstruction

4.10 Principles of Complex Reconstruction Planning

The mandibula is affected by neoplasms and osteoradionecrosis to a much greater extent than the maxilla. Substantial principles of lower jaw reconstructions with fibula flaps are representatively demonstrated in the following text. Special attention is paid to individually built and commercially available planning and osteotomy devices.

4.10.1 Classification of Mandibular Defects

Various classification schemes for mandibular defects have been suggested. Although the system after Jewer et al. (1989) is widespread, the classification after Urken et al. (1991) seems to have more impact on reconstruction planning. The lower jaw is divided as follows: C for condyle, R for ramus, B for body, and S for symphysis.

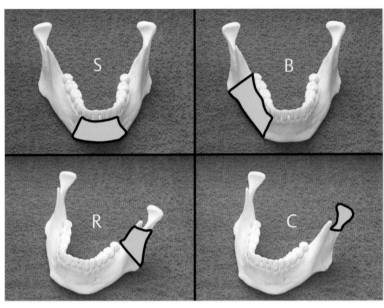

Fig. 4.76 Classification of mandibular defects after Urken et al. (1991). S, symphysis, from canine to canine; B, body, from canine to angle; R, ramus, from angle to incisura; C, condylar, from incisura to condyle.

4.10.2 Mandibular Reconstruction with Osseocutaneous Fibula Flaps

Reconstruction of the Basal Part or the Alveolar Process

Basal part reconstruction is recommended when mouth opening is reduced to less than 25 mm and consecutive insertion of dental implants is not possible.

Alveolar part reconstruction is recommended in patients with unrestricted mouth opening and possibility of consecutive dental implant insertion.

Choice of Donor Site for Osseocutaneous Fibula Flaps

The laterality of the fibula donor site depends on
• Whether the skin island is used for intraoral or extraoral reconstruction
• Whether the anastomoses are performed on the ipsi- or contralateral neck with respect to the fibula donor site

Anastomoses	Positioning of skin island	Laterality of fibula donor site
Left neck	Intraoral	Right fibula
Right neck	Intraoral	Left fibula
Left neck	Extraoral	Left fibula
Right neck	Extraoral	Right fibula

Fig. 4.77 Algorithm for osseocutaneous fibula harvest with respect to the location of anastomoses and soft tissue reconstruction.

Reconstruction of Class B Defects

Preoperative planning and operative management of an osteoradionecrosis case is demonstrated in Figs. 4.78 and 4.79. The patient underwent surgery and postoperative radiotherapy because of tongue cancer. Because of the intraoral dehiscence and the irradiated and insufficient cervical skin, a reconstructive procedure with two flaps was planned. An osseocutaneous fibula flap was suggested for mandibular and intraoral reconstruction with an additional radial forearm flap for extraoral coverage. Anastomoses for both flaps were to be performed on the contralateral, unoperated neck side. Due to the reduced mouth opening of the patient (15 mm preoperatively), the fibula transplant was placed at the mandibular base.

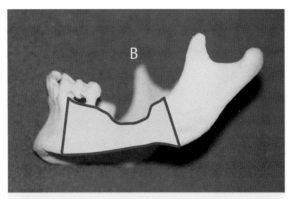

Fig. 4.79 Fabrication of a stereolithography (SLA) model from mandibula and fibula (not shown).

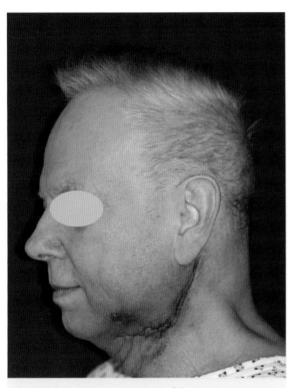

Fig. 4.78 Preoperative presentation of the patient.

Preoperative Manufacturing of Individualized Cutting Devices and Operation

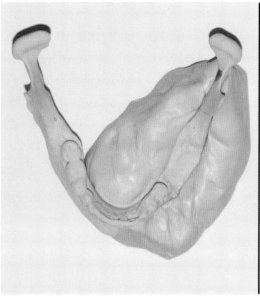
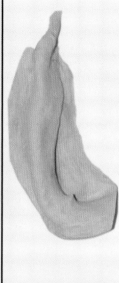

Fig. 4.80 Impression of the basal part of the mandible, which needs to be reconstructed, and construction of a plaster model.

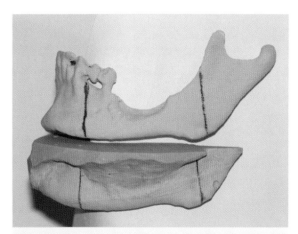

Fig. 4.81 Defining the resection.

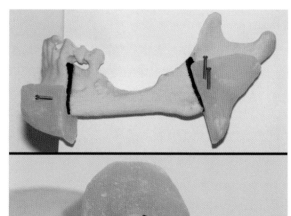

Fig. 4.82 Isolation of the plaster model. Individualized polymethyl methacrylate (PMMA) cutting guides with drilling holes are built.

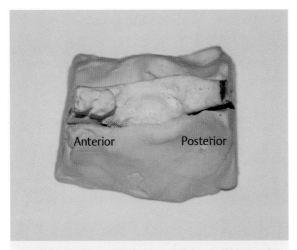

Fig. 4.83 Impression of the basal part of the mandible together with mandibular cutting guides. Defined resection of the diseased part of the mandible (on SLA model).

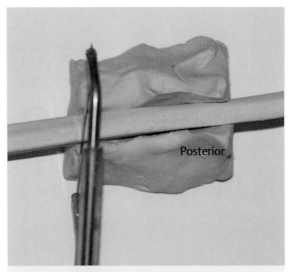

Fig. 4.84 According to the location of the perforator vessels, the SLA fibula is placed in the impression. Saw the fibula segment in accordance to the resection line.

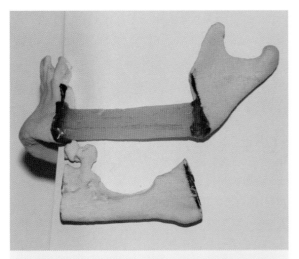

Fig. 4.85 The fibula segment is fixed with wax. If preoperative mouth opening is poor, as it is (15 mm), and dental implants will not be inserted, the fibula substitutes for the basal part of the mandibular body.

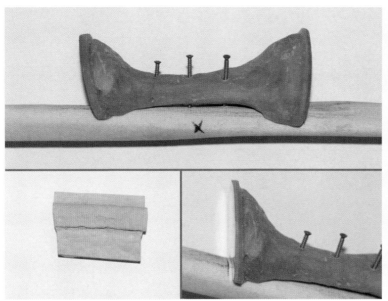

Fig. 4.86 Doubling the lateral rim of the fibular segment and fabrication of a plaster model. Fibular cutting guide is built from PMMA or an addition cross-linking silicone with respect to the location of the perforator. Drilling holes for fixation screws are prepared.

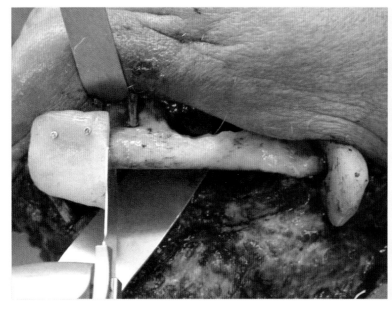

Fig. 4.87 PMMA cutting guides are fixed on the mandible.

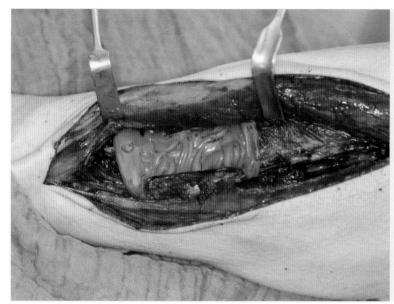

Fig. 4.88 Fixation of the silicone cutting guide on the fibula.

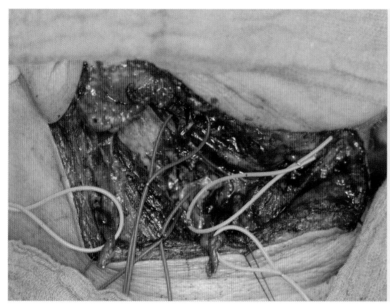

Fig. 4.89 Preparation of recipient vessels for radial forearm flap and fibula flap (arteries and veins) at the contralateral neck side.

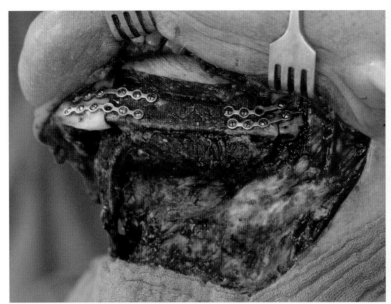

Fig. 4.90 Intraoperative status after anastomosis, insertion, and osteosynthesis of the fibula.

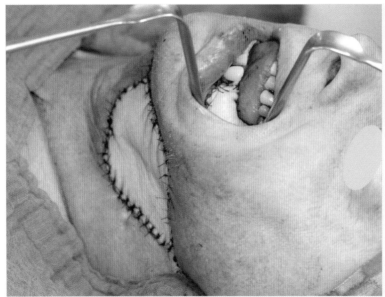

Fig. 4.91 Radial forearm flap and fibula flap at the end of the operation.

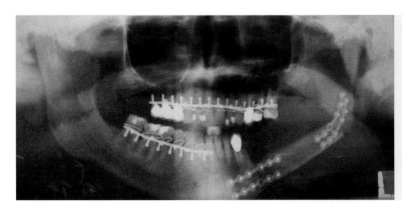

Fig. 4.92 Postoperative panoramic X-ray.

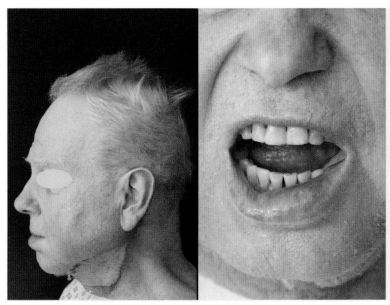

Fig. 4.93 Clinical view 12 days postoperatively.

Reconstruction of Class BR Defects

BR defects are characterized by a missing vertical reference. Thus, planning is performed with the commercially available virtual ProPlan CMF system (SYNTHES, Freiburg, Germany, and Materialise, Leuven, Belgium). After computed tomography (CT) of the head and neck region and the lower limb region resection of the mandibula, osteotomies of the fibula and reconstruction are simulated virtually. Corresponding cutting guides are fabricated. A case of a 49-year-old woman with a preoperative mouth opening of 41 mm is presented in Figs. 4.95 to 4.98.

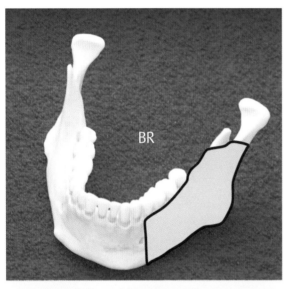

Fig. 4.94 Mandibular BR defect schematically.

Virtual Planning of Mandibular and Fibular Osteotomy (SYNTHES, Freiburg, Germany, and Materialise, Leuven, Belgium)

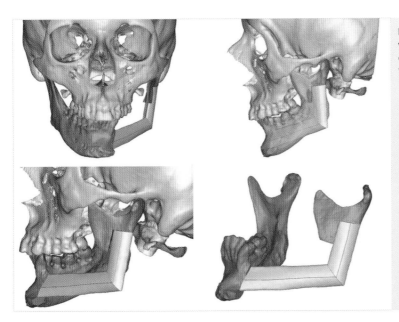

Fig. 4.95 After CT of mandible: virtual 3D visualization of the mandibular defect and determination of resection margins and fibula placement.

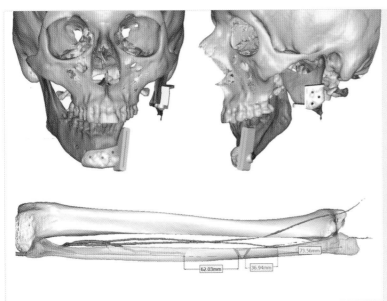

Fig. 4.96 Virtual placement of the mandibular cutting guides. Determination of the fibular osteotomies.

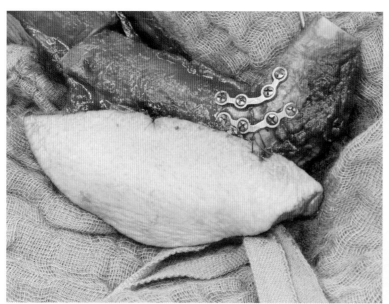

Fig. 4.97 Osteotomized and osteosynthe-sized fibular transplant.

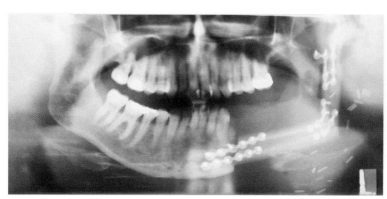

Fig. 4.98 Postoperative panoramic X-ray of the mandibular reconstruction. Fibula transplant is placed cranially.

Reconstruction of Class BSB Defects

Planning of BSB defects is performed virtually.

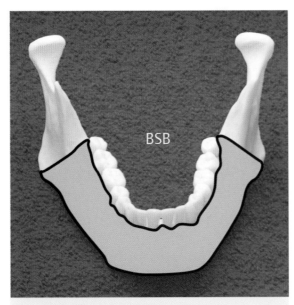

Fig. 4.99 Mandibular BSB defect schematically.

Cutting Devices Manufactured After Virtual Planning

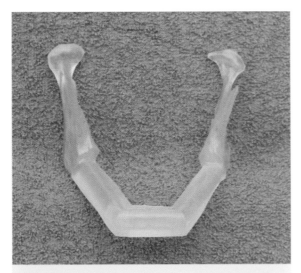

Fig. 4.100 CT-guided 3D reconstruction of the neo-mandible and fabrication of an SLA model.

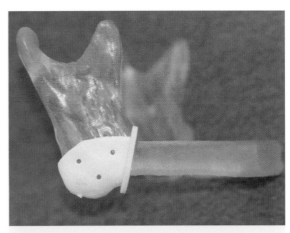

Fig. 4.101 Prefabricated cutting device for mandibular resection.

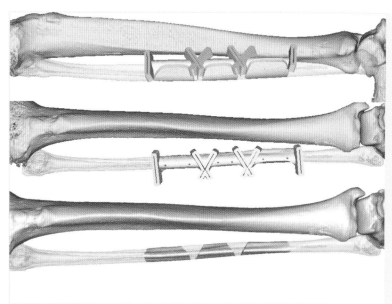

Fig. 4.102 Example of virtual adaptation and fabrication of fibular cutting guides (not case related).

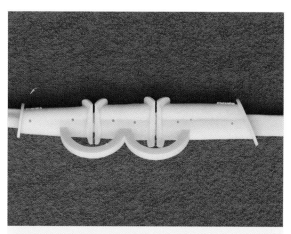

Fig. 4.103 Cutting guide placed on stereolithography model of the fibula.

Intraoperative Application

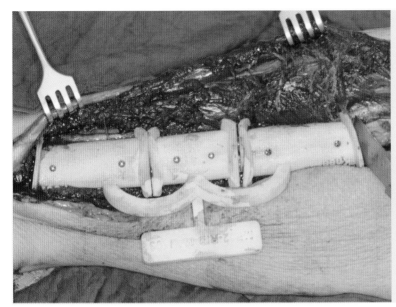

Fig. 4.104 Prefabricated cutting device for fibular osteotomies.

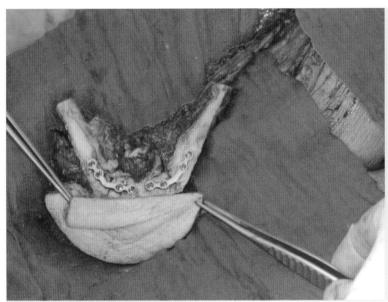

Fig. 4.105 From fibula to neo-mandible with skin island.

Modification: Osseous Fibula Transplant with Primary Implantation

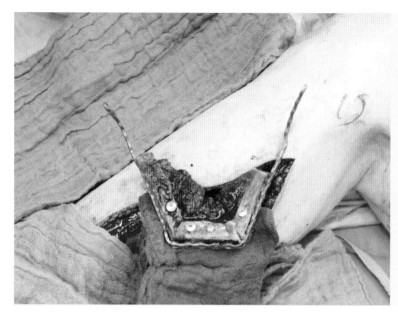

Fig. 4.106 Four dental implants are primarily inserted when flap is still pedicled.

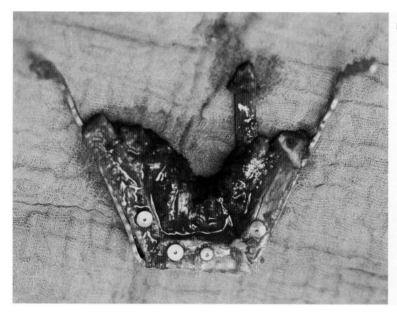

Fig. 4.107 Neo-mandible with implants.

Modification: Fibula Transplant with Two Skin Islands

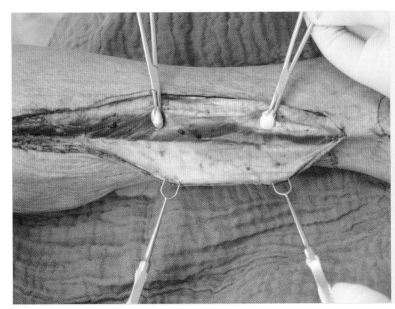

Fig. 4.108 Visualization of several skin perforators.

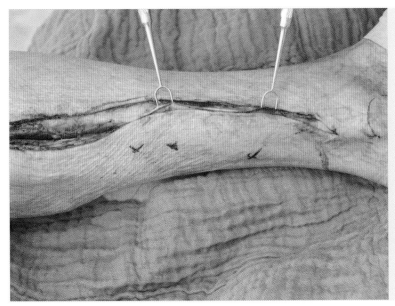

Fig. 4.109 Marking the perforators in the lateral skin region of the lower limb.

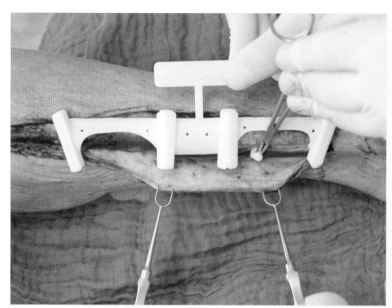

Fig. 4.110 Application of the cutting guide with respect to the perforators.

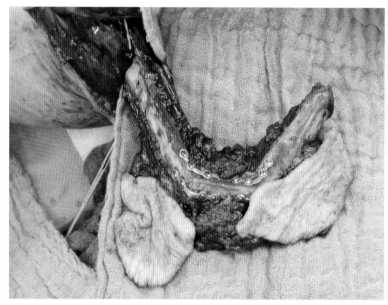

Fig. 4.111 Osteosynthesized neo-mandible with two skin paddles.

4.10.3 Combined Mandibula and Tongue Reconstruction

The operative management of an extended oral cancer case is presented in Figs. 4.112 to 4.118. The tumor mass infiltrated the tongue, the mandible, and the skin in the submental region. After tumor removal and neck dissection, the former tumor region was reconstructed by anterolateral thigh flap and an osseocutaneous fibula flap. Anastomoses for the anterolateral thigh flap were performed on the right neck, for the fibula flap on the left neck.

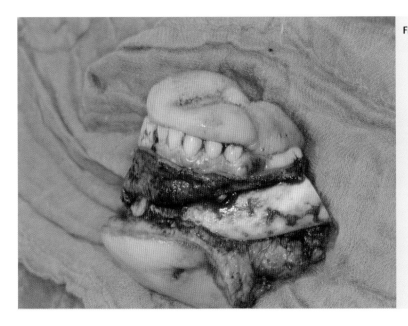

Fig. 4.112 Resected tumor mass.

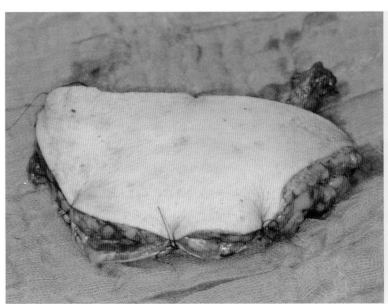

Fig. 4.113 Anterolateral thigh flap for tongue reconstruction is harvested.

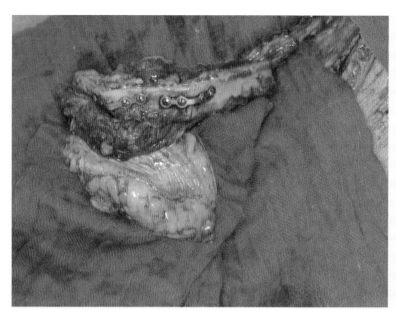

Fig. 4.114 Osseocutaneous fibula flap for mandibular and extraoral skin reconstruction is still pedicled at the lower limb. Fibula segments are osteotomized and osteosynthesized according to the cutting guides.

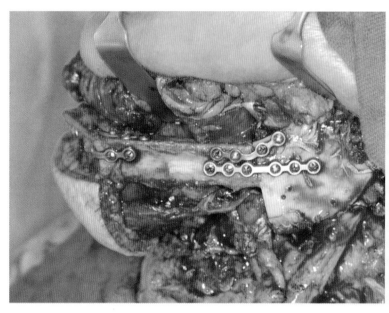

Fig. 4.115 Neo-mandible is anastomosed, inserted, and osteosynthesized. Skin paddle of the fibula flap in the submental region.

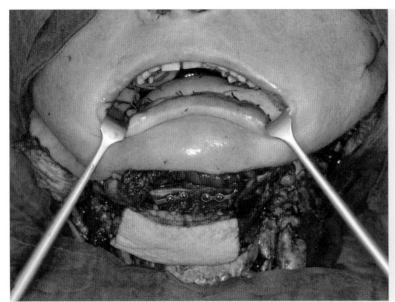

Fig. 4.116 Anterior view: anterolateral thigh flap is also anastomosed and covers the intraoral defect region.

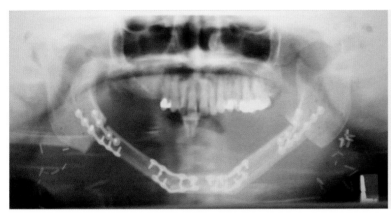

Fig. 4.117 Panoramic X-ray 10 days post-operatively. Bony reconstruction follows the cranial rim of the mandible.

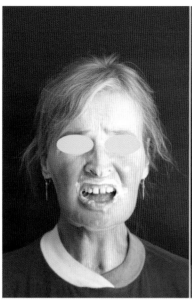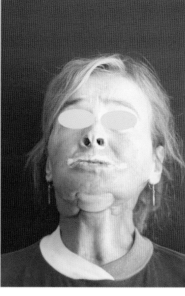

Fig. 4.118 Patient 10 weeks after operation while receiving postoperative radiotherapy.

Recommended Reading

Aymard JL. Nasal reconstruction. With a note on nature's plastic surgery. Lancet 1917; 2: 888–892

Bakamjian VY. A two-stage method for pharyngooesophageal reconstruction with a primary pectoral skin flap. Plast Reconstr Surg 1965; 36: 173–184

Biemer E, Stock W. Total thumb reconstruction: a one-stage reconstruction using an osteo-cutaneous forearm flap. Br J Plast Surg 1983; 36: 52–55

Carrel A. La technique opératoire des anastomoses vasculaires et la transplantation des viscères. Lyon Med 1902; 98: 859–865

Carrel A. Results of the Transplantation of Blood Vessels, Organs and Limbs. JAMA 1908; 51: 1662–1667

Dieffenbach JF. Chirurgische Erfahrungen besonders über die Wiederherstellung zerstörter Theile des menschlichen Körpers nach neuen Methoden. Berlin: T.C.F. Enslin; 1829–1834

Esser JFS. Deckung von Gaumendefekten mittels gestielter Naso-Labial-Hautlappen. Dtsch Zeitschr Chir. 1918; 147: 128–135

Hidalgo DA. Fibula free flap: a new method of mandible reconstruction. Plast Reconstr Surg 1989; 84: 71–79

Hill HL, Nahai F, Vasconez LO. The tensor fascia lata myocutaneous free flap. Plast Reconstr Surg 1978; 61: 517–522

Jacobson JH, Suarez EL: Microsurgery in anastomosis of small vessels. Surg Forum 1960; 11: 243–245

Jassinowsky A. Die Arteriennaht: eine experimentell-chirurgische Studie. Dorpat: Mattiesen; 1889

Jewer DD, Boyd JB, Manktelow RT et al. Orofacial and mandibular reconstruction with the iliac crest free flap: a review of 60 cases and a new method of classification. Plast Reconstr Surg 1989; 84: 391–403, discussion 404–405

Kesting MR, Hölzle F, Wolff KD et al. Use of microvascular flap technique in older adults with head and neck cancer: a persisting dilemma in reconstructive surgery? J Am Geriatr Soc 2011; 59: 398–405

Kimura N, Satoh K. Consideration of a thin flap as an entity and clinical applications of the thin anterolateral thigh flap. Plast Reconstr Surg 1996; 97: 985–992

Krag C, Kirkby B. The deltopectoral flap: a historical review with comments on its role in neurovascular reconstruction. Scand J Plast Reconstr Surg 1980; 14: 145–150

McLean DH, Buncke HJ. Autotransplant of omentum to a large scalp defect, with microsurgical revascularization. Plast Reconstr Surg 1972; 49: 268–274

Mühlbauer W, Herndl E, Stock W. The forearm flap. Plast Reconstr Surg 1982; 70: 336–344

Nahai F, Silverton JS, Hill HL, Vasconez LO. The tensor fascia lata musculocutaneous flap. Ann Plast Surg 1978; 1: 372–379

Nahai F, Hill L, Hester TR. Experiences with the tensor fascia lata flap. Plast Reconstr Surg 1979; 63: 788–799

Schmidt BL, Dierks EJ. The nasolabial flap. Oral Maxillofac Surg Clin North Am 2003; 15: 487–495, v

Seidenberg B, Hurwitt ES. Immediate reconstruction of the cervical esophagus by a revascularized isolated jejunal segment. Surg Forum 1958; 9: 413–416

Seidenberg B, Rosenak SS, Hurwitt ES, Som ML. Immediate reconstruction of the cervical esophagus by a revascularized isolated jejunal segment. Ann Surg 1959; 149: 162–171

Song YG, Chen GZ, Song YL. The free thigh flap: a new free flap concept based on the septocutaneous artery. Br J Plast Surg 1984; 37: 149–159

Soutar DS, Scheker LR, Tanner NS, McGregor IA. The radial forearm flap: a versatile method for intra-oral reconstruction. Br J Plast Surg 1983; 36: 1–8

Stock W, Mühlhauer W, Biemer E. Der neurovaskuläre Unterarm-Insel-Lappen [The neurovascular forearm island flap]. Z Plast Chir 1981; 5: 158–165

Taylor GI, Miller GD, Ham FJ. The free vascularized bone graft. A clinical extension of microvascular techniques. Plast Reconstr Surg 1975; 55: 533–544

Urken ML, Weinberg H, Vickery C, Buchbinder D, Lawson W, Biller HF. Oromandibular reconstruction using microvascular composite free flaps. Report of 71 cases and a new classification scheme for bony, soft-tissue, and neurologic defects. Arch Otolaryngol Head Neck Surg 1991; 117: 733–744

Von Langenbeck B. Ueber eine neue Methode der totalen Rhinoplastik. Berl Klin Wchnschr. 1864; 1: 13–14

Wei FC, Chen HC, Chuang CC, Noordhoff MS. Fibular osteoseptocutaneous flap: anatomic study and clinical application. Plast Reconstr Surg 1986; 78: 191–200

Wei FC, Jain V, Celik N, Chen HC, Chuang DC, Lin CH. Have we found an ideal soft-tissue flap? An experience with 672 anterolateral thigh flaps. Plast Reconstr Surg 2002; 109: 2219–2226, discussion 2227–2230

Wolff KD, Grundmann A. The free vastus lateralis flap: an anatomic study with case reports. Plast Reconstr Surg 1992; 89: 469–475, discussion 476–477

Yang G, Chen B, Gao Y et al. Forearm free skin flap transplantation. Natl Med J China. 1981; 61: 139–141

Zlotolow IM, Huryn JM, Piro JD, Lenchewski E, Hidalgo DA. Osseointegrated implants and functional prosthetic rehabilitation in microvascular fibula free flap reconstructed mandibles. Am J Surg 1992; 164: 677–681

Index

A

Ablative tumor surgery, 33–49
– access to tumor in, 34
–– overview and accessibility, 34
–– alternative approaches and indications for, 34
– Le Fort I osteotomy approach for, 46-47
–– history of, 46
–– technique of, 46–47
– lip-split mandibulotomy access for, 34–40
–– history of, 34
–– modifications of, 35
–– technique of, 36–40
–– midfacial degloving for, 43–45
–– history of, 43
–– technique of, 43–45
– Weber-Fergusson-Dieffenbach approach for, 41–42
–– history of, 41
–– technique of, 41–42
– tumor access, further approaches for, 47
– tumor resection, 48–49
Airway management. See Tracheotomy
Algorithms for reconstructive surgery, 52–53
Allen, Edgar Van Nuys, 70
Allen test, 70
Alveolar process of mandible, reconstruction of, 98
Anterior iliac crest bone flap, 96
Anterolateral thigh flap/myocutaneous vastus lateralis flap, 75–84
– with additional myocutaneous tensor fasciae latae flap, 83–84
– anatomic landmarks in, 75–76
– for combined mandibular and tongue reconstruction, 115–118
– history of, 75
– incision for, 77
– indication for, 75
– preoperative procedures for, 75
– technique of, 75–82
Archer, Daniel, 46
Asclepiades, 2
ASIS (anterior superior iliac spine) in anterolateral thigh flap/myocutaneous vastus lateralis flap, 75–76
Aymard, J. L., 60

B

"Bakamjian flap," 60
Bakamjian, Vahram, 60
Basal part of mandible, reconstruction of, 98
Belmont, Judson R., 46
Bier, August, 54

Bocca, Ettore, 10
Brassavola, Antonio Musa, 2
Bretonneau, Pierre, 2
Buncke, Harry, 66

C

Carrel, Alexis, 66
Cervical lymph node groups, 12–14
Cohen, James, 35
Conley modification of Schobinger approach, 32
Converse, John Marquis, 43
Cooper, Veronica, 43
Cricoid cartilage, 3
Crile, George Washington, 10
Cutting devices
– manufactured after virtual planning, 107–116
– preoperative manufacture of individualized, 100–103
– with virtual ProPlan CMF system, 107–116

D

Deep circumflex iliac artery flap, 96
Deltopectoral flap, 60–65
– design and anatomy of, 60
– first stage procedure for, 61–63
– history of, 60
– indication for, 61
– second stage procedure for, 64–65
Dental implants, 85, 98, 101, 112
Dieffenbach, Johann Friedrich, 41, 54
Double-Y incision of Martin, 32

E

Esser, Johannes F. S., 54

F

Fergusson, William, 41
Fibula flap, osseocutaneous. See Osseocutaneous fibula flap
Free flaps, 96

G

Galen, 2
Gao Yuzhi, 70

H

Handedness and radial forearm flap, 70
Hidalgo, David, 85
H incision, 32

I

"Indian forehead flap," 54
Infrahyoid region, 3

J

Jackson, Chevalier, 2
Jacobsen, Julius, 66
Jassinowsky, Alexander, 66
Jawdynski, Franciszek, 10
Jugular notch, 3, 4

L

Laryngeal prominence, 3, 4
Latissimus dorsi flap, 96
– microvascular reanastomosed, 96
Le Fort I osteotomy approach, 46–47
Lip-split mandibulotomy access, 34–40
– history of, 34
– modifications of, 35
– technique of, 36–40
Lower jaw defects, algorithm for closure of, 53
Lower jugular nodes, 13
Lymph node management. See Neck dissection

M

MacFee approach for levels IV and V neck dissection, 25, 27–30
Mandibular defects
– class B after Urken, 99–105
– class BR after Urken, 106–108
– class BSB after Urken, 109–114, 116–117
– classification of, 97
Mandibular reconstruction with osseocutaneous fibula flap, 98–114
– algorithm for, 98
– of basal part or alveolar process, 98
– choice of donor site for, 98
– for class B defects after Urken, 99–105
– for class BR defects after Urken, 106–108
– for class BSB defects after Urken, 109–114, 116–117
– combined tongue and, 115–118
– cutting devices manufactured after virtual planning in, 107–116
– preoperative manufacturing of individualized cutting devices for, 100–103, 107–116
– with primary implantation, 112

– and radial forearm flap, 99, 104 - 105
– with two skin islands, 113–114
– virtual planning of mandibular and fibular osteotomy in, 107–108
Mandibulotomy access, lip-split, 34–40
– history of, 34
– modifications of, 35
– technique of, 36–40
McGregor, Ian, 35
McLean, Donald, 66
Microvascular anastomosis, 66–69
Middle jugular nodes, 13
Midfacial degloving, 43–45
Modified Schobinger approach for neck dissection, 25, 31
Mühlbauer, Wolfgang, 70
Myocutaneous tensor fasciae latae flap, 83–84
Myocutaneous vastus lateralis flap. See Anterolateral thigh flap/myocutaneous vastus lateralis flap

N

Nahai, Foad, 83
Nasolabial flap, 54–59
– anatomy of, 54
– history of, 54
– indications for, 55
– technique for, 55–59
– variations on, 55
Neck dissection, 9–32
– bilateral, 10
– cervical lymph node groups in, 12–14
– classification and clinical management of, 10
– en bloc resection in, 10
– general overview of, 10–14
– history of, 10
– ipsilateral, 10
– levels I to III (supraomohyoid), 15–24
– levels IV and V, 25–30
–– alternative approaches for, 31–32
– modified radical, 10
– radical, 10
– relevant anatomy for, 11
Neo-mandible, 85, 109, 111, 112, 114, 116

O

Obwegeser, Hugo, 46
Osseocutaneous fibula flap, 85–95
– contraindication for, 85
– cross-sectional anatomy for, 87
– history of, 85
– indication for, 85, 86

– mandibular reconstruction with, 98–118
–– algorithm for, 98
–– of basal part or alveolar process, 98
–– choice of donor site for, 98
–– for class B defects after Urken, 99–105
–– for class BR defects after Urken, 106–108
–– for class BSB defects after Urken, 109–114, 116–117
–– combined tongue and, 115–118
–– cutting devices manufactured after virtual planning in, 100–103, 107–116
–– preoperative manufacturing of individualized cutting devices for, 100–103, 107–116
–– with primary implantation, 112
–– and radial forearm flap, 99, 103, 104
–– with two skin islands, 113–114
–– virtual planning of mandibular and fibular osteotomy in, 100–103, 107–116
– preoperative procedures for, 85
– technique of, 88–95

P

Pectoralis major flap, 96
Pedicled flaps, 96
Posterior approach for levels IV and V neck dissection, 25, 27–30
Posterior triangle group, 14
ProPlan CMF system, 106–108

R

Radial forearm flap, 70–74
– Allen test for, 70

– as soft tissue substitute for class B mandibular defects after Urken, 99, 103, 104
– handedness and, 70
– history of, 70
– indication for, 70
– technique for, 71–74
Reconstructive surgery, 51–118
– algorithms for, 52–53
– anterolateral thigh flap/myocutaneous vastus lateralis flap in, 75–84
–– history of, 75
–– indication for, 75
–– modification by harvesting additional myocutaneous tensor fasciae latae flap in, 83–84
–– preoperative procedures for, 75
–– technique of, 75–82
– classification of mandibular defects for, 97
– complex, 97–118
– considerations on, 52
– deltopectoral flap in, 60–65
– free flaps in, 96
– mandibular with osseocutaneous fibula flaps, 98–114
–– of basal part or alveolar process, 98
–– choice of donor site for, 98
–– for class B defects after Urken, 99–105
–– for class BR defects after Urken, 106–108
–– for class BSB defects after Urken, 109–114, 116–117
–– combined tongue and, 115–118
– microvascular anastomosis in, 66–69
– nasolabial flap in, 54–59
– osseocutaneous fibula flap in, 85–95
–– contraindication for, 85

–– cross-sectional anatomy for, 87
–– history of, 85
–– indication for, 85, 86
–– preoperative procedures for, 85
–– technique of, 88–95
– pedicled flaps in, 96
– radial forearm flap in, 70–74
Robson, Martin, 35
Roux, Philibert Joseph, 34, 35

S

Sasaki, Clarence T., 46
Scapular flap, 96
Schobinger approach
– Conley modification of, 32
– modified, 25, 31
Seidenberg, Bernard, 66
Single-Y incision, 32
SLA (stereolithography) model, 99–102, 109, 110
Soft tissue defect coverage, algorithm for, 52
Soutar, David, 70
Stereolithography (SLA) model, 99–102, 109, 110
Suarez, Ernesto, 66
Suarez, Osvaldo, 10
Submandibular nodes, 12
Submandibular triangle, 12
Submental nodes, 12
Submental triangle, 12
Supraomohyoid dissection, 15–24
– local anesthesia for, 16
– patient positioning for, 16
– preliminary considerations and recommended procedure for, 15
– technique of, 16–24
Sushruta, 54

T

Taylor, Ian, 85

–– cross-sectional anatomy for, 87

Temporalis muscle flap, 96
Tensor fasciae latae (TFL) flap, myocutaneous, 83–84
Tongue reconstruction, combined mandibular and, 115–118
Tracheal tube, 8
Tracheotomy, 1–8
– history of, 2
– relevant anatomy for, 3
– technique of, 4–8
Trousseau, Armand, 2
Tumor resection, 48–49

U

Upper jaw defects, algorithm for closure of, 53
Upper jugular nodes, 12
Uttley, David, 46

V

Vastus lateralis (VL) flap, myocutaneous. See Anterolateral thigh flap/myocutaneous vastus lateralis flap
Virtual ProPlan CMF system, 107–117
von Graefe, Albrecht, 34
von Langenbeck, Bernhard, 46, 54

W

Washington, George, 2
Weber-Fergusson-Dieffenbach approach, 41–42
Weber, Karl Otto, 41

Y

Yang Guofan, 70